Occupational Therapy and the Patient with Pain

Occupational Therapy and the Patient with Pain

Florence S. Cromwell
Editor

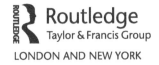

Routledge
Taylor & Francis Group

LONDON AND NEW YORK

First Published 1984 by The Haworth Press, Inc.

Published 2014 by Routledge
711 Third Avenue, New York, NY 10017 USA
2 Park Square, Milton Park, Abingdon, Oxon OX14 4RN

Routledge is an imprint of the Taylor & Francis Group, an informabusiness

Occupational Therapy and the Patient with Pain has also been published as *Occupational Therapy in Health Care,* Volume 1, Number 3, Fall 1984.

Reprint - 2007

Library of Congress Cataloging in Publication Data
Main entry under title:

Occupational therapy and the patient with pain.

"Has also been published as Occupational therapy in health care, volume 1, number 3, fall 1984"—T.p. verso.
    Includes bibliographical references.
    1. Pain—Treatment—Addresses, essays, lectures. 2. Intractable pain—Treatment—Addresses, essays, lectures. 3. Occupational therapy—Addresses, essays, lectures.
I. Cromwell, Florence S. [DNLM: 1. Pain—rehabilitation. 2. Palliative Treatment.
3. Occupational Therapy. W1 0C601H v.1 no.3 / WB 555 0142]
RB127.023 1984   616'.0472   84-10496
ISBN 0-86656-306-7

ISBN 978-1-315-86419-8 (eISBN)

Occupational Therapy and the Patient with Pain

Occupational Therapy in Health Care
Volume 1, Number 3

CONTENTS

FROM THE EDITOR'S DESK   **1**

**FROM ANOTHER PERSPECTIVE: A CLINICIAN'S
VIEW OF THE THEME**   **3**
  Janice S. Matsutsuyu

Occupational Therapy and the Patient with Pain   **7**
  Jerry A. Johnson

  Pain Defined   8
  Characteristics and Consequences of Pain   10
  Approaches to Treatment   11
  Treatment Programs: The Health Care Team   12
  Occupational Therapy   13

**Stress Management as a Component of Occupational
Therapy in Acute Care Settings**   **17**
            Anne Affleck
            Elizabeth Bianchi
            Marlene Cleckley
            Karen Donaldson
            Guy McCormack
            Jan Polon

  Stress—Components and Responses   18
  Interventions   20
  Program Models   22

Chronic Pain   37
Summary   39

Occupational Therapy Intervention in Chronic Pain   **43**
  Anne B. Blakeney

Chronic Pain Syndrome   44
Secondary Problems   44
Causes   45
The Gate Control Theory   46
Treatment   48
Occupational Therapy Intervention   50
Case Vignette   50
Conclusion   53

Perspectives on the Pain of the Hospice Patient:
The Roles of the Occupational Therapist and Physician   **55**
  Kent Nelson Tigges
  Lawrence Mark Sherman
  Frances S. Sherwin

Biological Pain   56
Management of Biological Pain   57
Pain of Isolation   58
Pain of Abandonment   59
The Hospice Philosophy   59
Pain of Loss of Role: The Role of Occupational Therapy   60
The Occupational Therapy Assessments   62
Case Study 1   63
Case Study 2   65
Conclusion   66

The Schultz Structured Interview for Assessing Upper
Extremity Pain   **69**
  Karen S. Schultz

Development of the Tool   71
Preparation for the Interview   72
Administration of the Assessment   72
The Interview Format   73
Summary   81

Shoulder Pain in the Patient with Hemiplegia:
A Fundamental Concern in Occupational Therapy   83
Charlotte Gowland

Occupational Therapist Impressions   84
Literature Review   84
Chart Review   85
Group Characteristics   86
Discussion   88
Unanswered Questions   90
Summary and Conclusions   90

The Role of Occupational Therapy in Back School   93
Joy White Randolph

Initial Treatment Plan   95
Results   96
Current Back School Plan   97
Results   99
Conclusion   101

The Use of Biofeedback Techniques in Occupational
Therapy for Persons with Chronic Pain   103
Shelley R. Rogers
Julie Shuer
Susan Herzig

The Chronic Pain Problem   104
Intervention   105
Outcomes   107
Summary   108

The Use of Assertiveness Training with Chronic Pain
Patients   109
Linda Lloyd Zelik

Problems Associated with the Chronic Pain Syndrome   110
Rationale for Using Assertiveness Training   111
Occupational Therapy's Role   111
Background   112
Advantages of Assertiveness   113
Description of Assertiveness Classes   113

Program Results and Case Examples   116
Conclusions   117

The Growth of the Hospice Movement: A Role
  for Occupational Therapy   **119**
              Pamela Brown

A Definition   120
A Look at the Beginnings—Britain   120
In the United States   122
Comparison   123
Kinds of Pain in Terminal Illness   123
Effects on Caregivers   125
Role of Occupational Therapy in Hospice   125
Conclusion   126

PRACTICE WATCH: THINGS TO THINK ABOUT

What Every Therapist Should Know: Hazards
  in the Clinic   **129**
              Michele Watkins
              Lawanna Drake
              Suzanne May

Chemicals   129
Ceramic Supplies   132
Fibers   133
Stress   133
Summary   134
Note   134

JANET C. STONE, BA, OTR, *Former Department Head, Occupational Therapy, Rancho Los Amigos Hospital, Downey, California, and Initiating Editor, AOTA Bulletin on Practice, Huntington Beach, CA*

CARL SUNDSTROM, MA, OTR, LTC, AMSC, *Occupational Therapy Staff Officer, Health Services Command, Fort Sam Houston, TX*

MARY GRACE WASHBURN, MHA, OTR, FAOTA, *Marketing Director, Health Care Design Services, Kirkham, Michael and Associates, Architects, Engineers and Planners, Denver, Colorado*

CARLOTTA WELLES, MA, OTR, FAOTA, *Consultant, Professional Liability, and Former Chairman, Occupational Therapy Department, Los Angeles City College, Los Angeles, CA*

Occupational Therapy and the Patient with Pain

FROM THE EDITOR'S DESK

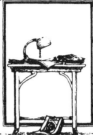

This the third issue of OTHC is the largest thus far in the short history of the journal. That it should focus on such a universal health and health care problem is doubtless related. There is much to be said about pain. Pain is certainly something we all have felt, for ourselves or with our patients, so with this issue we indeed speak to concerns of therapists in all areas of practice in this profession.

Only after we had begun to plan and solicit papers for this theme did it become apparent that occupational therapists are much involved with patients disabled by pain. So it is not *if* we are involved, but *how* and *why* occupational therapists are treating patients suffering from pain that become the critical questions to explore. These questions can be addressed at least in part through the papers here assembled.

The broad scope of the articles presented provides anyone with a better understanding of pain, its causes and effects. They also show any number of ways occupational therapists are addressing pain, how to relieve it, or live with it. Happily most of this is done in the context of the profession's philosophy to enhance individuals' abilities to carry out the activities so basic to role functioning.

Our hope is that the information you glean from reading the papers and discussing them with colleagues will help you respond to the challenge made by Matsutsuyu in her feature critique, concerning the relationship of this special area of current focus to the broad goals in treatment which the profession has affirmed. And to the need for us as a profession, in the midst of striking changes in health care delivery, to finally come to grips with what shall be the arena and scope of our practice.

This issue also inaugurates another feature with the appearance of *Practice Watch.* Intended as a vehicle for sharing ideas on topics of general concern, in this instance three young writers translated a student project from recent undergraduate days into an essay on a clinical question we all could well examine and heed.

The next, and final issue in Volume I, will turn to some of the most fundamental activities and interests of occupational therapy as it draws attention to the occupational therapist's particular interest and skill in facilitating adaptation for patients otherwise disabled in performance of their role activities. Be it through application of devices and equipment, teaching new or substitute behaviors or changing the environment, the authors to be included in the next issue will challenge you with their thinking and their solutions.

Florence S. Cromwell
Editor

FROM ANOTHER PERSPECTIVE:
A CLINICIAN'S VIEW
OF THE THEME

Who among us cannot recall faces of patients grimacing with pain, the anxieties with which we tentatively approached a fearful patient to actively engage in a task perceived as painful and how we sighed with relief when the patient said, "it wasn't that bad." Occupational therapy caseloads have always included and will continue to include patients with symptoms of pain or an array of behaviors associated with pain, whatever the diagnosis, etiology or course of illness.

That there is now effort which focuses on behavioral management of patients with chronic pain opens infinite possibilities that we in occupational therapy might act on. Especially that we might be able to further optimize, with more quality, a painful patient's ability to perform the tasks of daily living and for achieving satisfaction in life roles.

Chronic pain can be so debilitating, so seriously dysfunctional and of such duration that a person must stop working, and cannot do or enjoy what used to be done in the course of daily routines. The hope for such patients lies in the advancements in medical treatment, new technology and methods of managing pain. The challenge for occupational therapy is to learn in what ways we can significantly add to our skills and knowledge so that we can assist patients to gain skills which not only lessen the erosive effects brought on by pain but which will maximize functional capacities.

Enthusiasm can be seen in clinicians seeking more understanding

3

about the nature of pain and of behaviors associated with it. The diversity of the articles in this issue offers an excellent opportunity for us to examine the state of the art in pain management and, in particular, what we are doing about it in occupational therapy. The articles range in focus from overviews of pain behaviors by Johnson and Blakeney to selected approaches for pain management by Rogers et al, Zelik and Randolph. Assessment of pain for specificity are proposed by Schultz and Gowland. The humanization of attitudes and environment for compassionately easing the discomfort of pain and to refocus energies toward gaining a sense of self-affirmation and competence by patients are valuable dimensions by Tigges et al, Johnson, Brown, Blakeney and Affleck et al.

Two intriguing articles illustrate how knowing more about pain, the behaviors associated with it and the application of pain management approaches can facilitate occupational therapy objectives to assist patients to become more functional in daily activities and for role satisfaction. Blakeney places knowledge about pain behaviors and a model of pain management in the context of an occupational therapy program based on a frame of reference from our discipline. It thereby differentiates the contributions of occupational therapy care and treatment of a patient with pain as distinct from other disciplines.

Affleck et al demonstrate the usefulness of one mode of approach. The applied principles of stress management and its various aspects are used to help patients with chronic pain, as well as other diagnoses, to achieve occupational therapy objectives for the patient. Both articles reflect commitment that the primary purpose of occupational therapy is to maximize the capabilities of patients to function so that they can go on with some, if not all aspects of their daily routines and role expectations.

This issue as a whole reflects the typical inclinations of occupational therapy to tackle difficult problems and to be open to new ideas. Undoubtedly new ways of helping patients can enrich our practice. But at the same time there is inherent risk in readily accepting popular trends for they may lead us astray unless we pay conscious attention to relevance of the new ideas and methods in the context of occupational therapy's purposes as a service for patients.

The question in my mind, in the form of a challenge, is whether or not the various means of treating, assessing and educating patients to manage or to live with the dysfunctions brought on by chronic pain will help and facilitate occupational therapy goals for the patient or if they will become treatment of choice in and of themselves. We have already experienced the divisiveness over modalities, i.e., heat and massage, the abandonment of crafts, the indiscriminate use of well founded testing such as the S.I. battery across the board of diagnosis and age groups, and the disarray in psychiatric occupational therapy because we cannot make up our minds whether we are occupational therapists or psychotherapists. Since readers will be able to cite example after example, we should be especially thankful that the authors of the articles in this issue give us the opportunity to study and openly discuss what we envision as future directions in this area of practice.

The issue on the theme of pain points to the need to know more about behaviors associated with pain, ways to discriminate various forms pain takes and offers possibilities for adding to our repertoire of existing skills for working with patients with pain. What needs further explication is what we as occupational therapists are going to do about it.

Future directions will most obviously be related to outcome studies of what will be beneficial vis à vis occupational therapy treatment for patients. These studies may also identify educational needs for continuing and entry level education. Furthermore, a realistic appraisal of what services will be reimbursed would be timely inasmuch as pain programs in general are having difficulties with payment by third party payors.

Most importantly, the sneak preview of this issue highlighted for one reactor an age old question about relevance of new trends in health care to occupational therapy practice and how we determine what we accept and promote as part of our objectives in the service of treating patients. The selection of what should guide studies and critiques of innovations is a professional responsibility which we are often reluctant to accept.

A start for guiding further directions in practice can be found in the American Occupational Therapy Association statement of occupational therapy definitions and functions. This is the statement of the fundamental purpose of occupational therapy as being that of "the development and maintenance of a persons's capacities through life, to perform with satisfaction to self and others those tasks and roles essential to productive living and the mastery of self and the environment."[1, pp 204]

---

[1]Occupational Therapy: Its Definitions and Functions. Am J Occup Ther, 26:4, 1972.

A concerted effort should yield many possibilities for more sound attention to a common condition called pain, be it transitory or chronic in nature.

Janice S. Matsutsuyu, MA, OTR, FAOTA
Chief, Rehabilitation Services
Neuropsychiatric Institute
University of California at Los Angeles

Occupational Therapy
and the Patient with Pain

Jerry A. Johnson, EdD, OTR, FAOTA

ABSTRACT. The characteristics, implications, consequences and costs of pain, particularly the chronic benign pain syndrome, are presented, and current approaches to treatment are briefly discussed. Contributions which occupational therapists are uniquely qualified to offer are described.

Occupational therapists are grounded in the concepts that mind, body and spirit are integrally related and that the patient must participate actively in the planning and implementation of any treatment program. The occupational therapist is a specialist in role functions and is skilled in assisting clients to plan and re-create structure for their lives that has been lost by virtue of their illness, disability, or pain.

The occupational therapist provides an environmental laboratory in which people can experiment with new behaviors and attitudes to restructure and regain control of their lives and to reestablish hope, competence, confidence and success as part of their daily activities. These concepts are basic to the successful treatment of the patient with chronic benign pain syndrome.

". . . pain disturbs all aspects of a person's life. Chronic pain is a disease whose symptoms may include the development of a stress-related illness; the stress of constant worry may aggravate an ulcer precipitated by alcoholism in a vulnerable individual. Pain changes the personality, erodes self-esteem and confidence, strains the bonds of family relations, and depresses the mood . . . the stress of living in pain overwhelms the individual and his environment."[1, p 83]

Jerry A. Johnson is President and Director, The Resource Center for Health and Well-Being, Inc., 234 Steele Street, Denver, Colorado 80206.

Pain has been identified by the directors of the Association for Research in Nervous and Mental Diseases as "the most pressing health problem facing Americans in the 1980's."[1,p5] Approximately 40 million Americans suffer from various forms of chronic pain. In 1981 the cost of compensating pain sufferers was estimated to be $20 billion dollars, and the cost of lost productivity increased the cost to $50 billion dollars.

While these statistics are awesome, they fail to express or convey the impact that chronic pain has upon the lives of those whom it affects. The structure of life is abandoned as "chronic pain *becomes* the disease and in its wake brings a new and potentially devastating array of health problems . . ."[1, p 2] Emotional stability and social structure are stripped away as the patient with chronic pain seeks to cope with and control his pain.

This paper will define pain by describing major types of pain and examining characteristics and consequences of pain for the patient. Chronic pain, and particularly the chronic benign pain syndrome, will be discussed in greater detail as its consequences for patients are devastating. Because chronic pain affects most facets of a patient's life, the occupational therapist must understand the dynamics of chronic pain and the experience of the patient who lives with chronic pain.

Finally, the approaches to treatment of chronic benign pain will be briefly explored, and the paper will conclude with a section on occupational therapy for patients with pain.

PAIN DEFINED

Throughout history pain has been a perplexing phenomenon, often associated with punishment. In fact, the word pain comes from the Latin word poena which means punishment. Perception of pain is influenced by many things, including early learning experiences; ethnic, cultural, and economic factors; birth experience, gender, sibling order, and age; right- or left-handedness; and frame of mind and environment.[2, p 57]

Pain is a highly integrated, multifaceted phenomenon[2, p 58] and is thought to have several complex components, including perception, emotion, cognition, and motivation. The perception of pain is accompanied by anxiety, anger, resentment, depression, and other emotions.[2, p 57] Cognition communicates the message that something is wrong and that the pain will continue unabated until the message is heeded. This process motivates the patient to seek relief or to take other action.

Smoller and Schulman describe pain as the body's way of communicating with the mind. It becomes an internal communication and the most common complaint that brings a patient to a doctor.[1, p 2] As a form of communication, acute pain warns one that there is need for rest and protection to promote healing. Chronic pain conveys other messages, many of which are complex and not readily understood by either the patient who experiences chronic pain or by the staff who work with the patient. Comprehending and understanding the messages of chronic pain requires careful documentation by the patient and a close working relationship with members of the health care team.

There are three major types of pain: acute pain, chronic malignant pain, and chronic benign pain. Acute pain requires immediate attention, is usually finite, and can be treated on a short-term basis by the use of medication, massage, or heat. Chronic malignant pain is usually associated with cancer and may be treated by surgical procedures, drugs, and/or narcotics. Chronic benign pain, which serves no useful purpose, persists. Rather than warning one of danger that needs attention, it becomes the damaged part.[1, p 34] Chronic pain has origins, such as physical injuries, emotional depression, or behavioral dysfunction or problems, but it also becomes a *process:* "a regulatory force influencing the course and conduct of an individual's life".[1, p 2] In essence, the original cause of pain no longer exists, yet the pain persists and assumes a life of its own separate from the original source.

Some patients with chronic pain report that they experience feelings of helplessness, worthlessness, hopelessness, futility and lethargy. Other patients experience feelings of tension, agitation, anxiety, and hypersensitivity. Excessive stimulation cannot be shut out, and environmental input produces bodily aches that are excruciatingly painful. Some persons alternate between these two emotional experiences associated with pain whereas others may experience both at the same time.[2, pp 65-66]

The search for a cause of chronic pain is most frequently futile, for the original source no longer exists. This contributes to the patient's dilemma, for he is then confronted with trying to accept and explain his pain when no reason for its existence can be identified.

CHARACTERISTICS AND CONSEQUENCES OF PAIN

The experience of chronic pain and the patient's inability to explain its cause, often lead to withdrawal, loneliness, isolation, avoidance of others, activity restrictions, a loss of structure in life, impaired coping ability, a time-warped and distorted perspective of life, and self-absorption which both blurs the boundaries of reality and distorts one's judgment.[1, p 8]

Obviously, chronic pain is destructive to individuals who experience it. However, it also is costly to society, as demonstrated by some of the following statistics.

> Five million people are disabled by low back pain and will pay $1.5 billion in hospital and doctor bills including 200,000 surgical procedures and nearly 19 million visits to doctors.
> The average American loses two weeks of productivity per year due to pain.
> Over $1 billion in over-the-counter pain medications are sold each year.
> Each year $400 million in the habit forming enormously addictive drug propoxythene are sold.[2, p 5]

From the patient's perspective therapy is often ineffective, sometimes destructive, and very costly. "The average chronic pain patient has had medical and surgical expenses ranging from $50,000 to $100,000 . . . only thirty-nine percent of workmen's compensation patients who have suffered back injuries return to work."[3, p 2]

Employers are often antagonistic to employees with work injuries, and the person who has been devastated by pain is often forced to perform jobs which are more difficult than those previously held.[3, p 3] This may lead to a resignation or a termination for poor job performance, thereby avoiding the costs of medical retirement.

The Mayo Clinic, which has worked with a large number of patients with chronic pain, identifies the following characteristics as representative of a typical patient. The person:

1. has had pain for a minimum of 7 years;
2. has low back pain;
3. has been hospitalized for a minimum of *six* times for pain related conditions;
4. has been operated on at least twice, generally with little, if any, improvement;

5. has pervasively and decisively failed to respond to any form of conservative medical treatment;
6. has not worked in two years and rarely, if ever, is the subject of work mentioned spontaneously in conversation, and
7. has been receiving compensation payments at sufficient levels to maintain a decent standard of living.[2, p 72]

In summary, neither the patient with chronic pain nor his family, employers, or others in his environment readily understand or accept the concept of pain when no basis for its existence can be identified. Consequently, the search for a cause becomes the patient's compelling motivator in life.

APPROACHES TO TREATMENT

The traditional and frequently unsuccessful approach to pain, and particularly to chronic benign pain, has been to treat the patient symptomatically rather than to consider the problem of pain as one with many facets. In other words, people are given drugs until symptoms are relieved without in-depth exploration of the process of pain or its meaning.

Pelletier writes that the study and treatment of chronic pain demonstrates the necessity of thinking of pain as a great teacher and of using it to achieve growth and change in one's life.[4, p 320] He believes this can best be accomplished within the context of holistic medicine, which recognizes the inextricable interaction between the person and his psychosocial environment. Mind and body function as an integrated unit, and *health exists* when they are in harmony.[4, p 12] From Pelletier's perspective pain conveys the message that the person with chronic pain is experiencing disharmony and needs to attend to that disharmony and its resulting conflict.

In some of the major pain treatment centers it is assumed that the primary process causing the pain in the individual is no longer correctable or curable and that pain relief is the only alternative left for handling the patient's complaint.[3, p 28]

To achieve this relief, several principles seem to contribute to successful treatment:

1. the patient's role in his own treatment is central to the success of the overall health care program;
2. pain must be understood as a uniquely human event; it is punishing and creates a multitude of health problems. Success-

ful pain control requires an understanding of persistent pain and the specific steps that may be taken to halt the progression; and

3. pain is a multisystem disorder affecting physical and psychological processes and is a learned maladaptive behavior reinforced by conditions, responses, ineffectual therapy, poor physical condition, the abuse and misuse of medication, emotional stress, anxiety, and poor nutrition.[1, pp 11-12]

Application of these principles is most successfully accomplished in treatment centers in which treatment approaches and plans are orchestrated and implemented in a holistic framework. For example, the treatment staff are concerned with the patient's medical condition; decreasing excessive drug use; and improving his nutritional and physical condition, communications and relationships, and activity levels.

Successful treatment also requires an active interaction among the patient, physicians, and other professionals involved in the total program of therapy.[1, p 70] Finally, recognition of the concept that pain carries a message requires pursuit of a treatment program that leads to understanding and alleviating or reducing pain by comprehending and understanding its message.

TREATMENT PROGRAMS: THE HEALTH CARE TEAM

Within this context treatment programs generally include a physical examination and complete medical history. Patients may be asked to describe their pain verbally as well as pictorially. To better understand pain and its relationship to the individual client, patients may also be asked to keep diaries for periods of time, such as 30 days, and to record information about their pain tolerance, medications, and relaxation patterns. They may be asked to complete pain questionnaires describing their pain, intellectual abilities, previous treatments, family relationships, using descriptive words that best describe their pain.

Record keeping actively involves patients in their therapy and makes them more responsible for being accurate as historians and for sharing specific forms of information with the physician that may get lost without written documentation. As patients see behavioral patterns they can take action to control their activities and the environmental and emotional situations that produce or reduce pain levels. This reduces some of the helplessness and tension that patients previously felt. For example, some patients initially report that their pain is constantly present. However, when they keep diaries and records they frequently find that their pain levels vary considerably. Sometimes they can even establish patterns that may show a relationship to time of day, certain events or emotions, or other factors. As this awareness increases they can become more responsible for their pain.

Early attempts are made to reduce the amount of medication that patients have been taking. Medication seldom reduces chronic pain; indeed, amounts required to produce any change increase rather rapidly and may lead to drug abuse or drug addiction. Furthermore, drugs interfere with the body's production of endorphins (which are believed to serve as natural pain relievers) and negatively affect mood and emotions.

Patients are encouraged, if not required, to engage in light physical exercise (such as walking or swimming) and to increase the amount of time and energy exerted in physical exercise.

Psychotherapy's value is somewhat uncertain although the use of goal directed groups has been very valuable. In these groups patients support each other in setting goals for themselves in terms of managing their pain, dealing more effectively with events and situations that exacerbate their pain, and restructuring their lives. Focus on pain itself is limited.

Another treatment approach is to improve communications. Family, friends, or roommates and where possible, employers, are involved as pain control is a function of the system, as well as a function of the individual with pain. Improved skill in communication is very valuable and may reduce the need for pain, in some patients.

Finally, nutrition must be considered. Physical activity and nutritional intake should be balanced and better patterns of eating need to be re-established.

OCCUPATIONAL THERAPY

The occupational therapist is highly qualified to be an integral part of the treatment program for patients with chronic pain. Philosophically, occupational therapists work with the "whole" patient—whose mind, spirit, and body are unified. Occupational therapists are also committed to working collaboratively with patients, who are viewed as primary members of the treatment team.

More specifically, occupational therapists are specialists in role behaviors. The chronic pain patient has frequently given up his role in almost every sphere of life (family, work, social, and community), has abandoned any semblance of structure in life, and has little sense of responsibility or feeling of control in life.

Given this breakdown in role behavior and function, the occupational therapist is in an ideal position to work with patients on their diaries, their activity logs, and other documents that enable the patients to document the courses of their pain, to examine the relation of pain to activity and relationships, and to identify patterns that will be helpful in understanding the messages of their pain.

Using knowledge of activities, structures, and roles, the occupational therapist can work with patients (using data from their diaries and logs) to re-establish daily schedules. A balance of exercise, nutrition, self-care, social activities, and avocations is importantly incorporated into the schedule.

Goal directed groups, in which patients support each other in establishing and carrying out goals for activities and structure are also part of occupational therapy. These groups can also be used to improve the level and quality of communications among patients and their families.

Groups, composed of patients and their families or friends, can be designed to work on projects requiring problem identification, solutions, decision-making, communications, and joint endeavors to complete a specified project. The occupational therapist observes the patterns of communication, relationships, and interactions and contributes to the process of reintegrating the patient into the family or other social environments by providing feedback on problematic interaction patterns.

Another major contribution the occupational therapist makes is to introduce patients to, and supervise their participation in, increasing levels of physical activity.

In all of these, as well as other treatment activities, the therapist seeks to empower patients to assume control and responsibility for their lives, thereby mastering their pain rather than being its slave.

In conclusion, the patient with chronic benign pain can influence the course of his pain, and can fulfill roles that make life meaningful. To this end, the occupational therapist is a valuable member of the pain program treatment team.

The occupational therapist provides an environmental laboratory in which people can experiment with new behaviors and attitudes to restructure and regain control of their lives and to reestablish hope, competence, confidence and success as part of their daily activities. These concepts are basic to the successful treatment of the patient with chronic benign pain syndrome.

REFERENCES

1. Smoller B, Schulman G: *Pain Control, The Bethesda Program,* Garden City, New York: Doubleday & Co., Inc., 1982
2. Bresler, DE: *Free Yourself From Pain,* New York: Simon and Schuster, 1979
3. Shealy CN: *The Pain Game,* Berkeley, California: Celestial Arts, 1976
4. Pelletier, KR: *Mind As Healer, Mind As Slayer,* New York: Dell Publishing Co., Inc., 1980

Stress Management as a Component of Occupational Therapy in Acute Care Settings

Anne Affleck, MS, OTR
Elizabeth Bianchi, OTR
Marlene Cleckley, BS, OTR
Karen Donaldson, OTR
Guy McCormack, MS, OTR
Jan Polon, BS, OTR

ABSTRACT. The recent explosion of stress literature in the medical community has created a new awareness of "stress" as a potentially destructive force in itself. Contributing to physical and psychological dysfunction, stress has now been linked with a wide range of diagnoses including cancer, cardiac disease and arthritis. The importance of incorporating stress management activities into daily life is increasingly apparent. Occupational therapists concerned with patients' ability to achieve health enhancing independent living skills are in a key position to help patients master stress management skills and incorporate them into activities of daily living. This article will explore the incorporation of stress management into occupational therapy programming for a variety of acute care patients. It will review the components of stress, the stress cycle, the relaxation response, the occupational therapy role based on a model of human occupation, and will review current programs through case study of four patients: one diagnosed with cancer (leukemia), one with anorexia nervosa, one with chronic pain and the fourth, a patient in medical intensive care.

Anne Affleck is Assistant Director of Physical and Occupational Therapy, Stanford University Hospital, Stanford, CA; Supervisor of Occupational Therapy; Part-time Instructor Occupational Therapy, San Jose State University. Elizabeth Bianchi is Staff Therapist, SUH; Graduate student, Occupational therapy, San Jose State University. Marlene Cleckley is Clinical Coordinator—Hoover Pavillion, SUH. Karen Donaldson is Staff Therapist, SUH; Graduate student, Occupational Therapy, San Jose State University. Guy McCormack is Assistant Professor, Occupational Therapy, San Jose State University; Relief Therapist, SUH; PhD Candidate. Jan Polon is Clinical Coordinator for Complex Case Teams, SUH.

17

One of the fundamental goals of occupational therapy at Stanford University Hospital is to enable patients to achieve effectiveness in the environment and mastery of life tasks. A concern for quality of life coupled with a sensitivity to the healing nature of purposeful activity has created in occupational therapy a focus on the use of activity to develop skills necessary for independent living and the management of meaningful life roles in work and leisure. But even in the context of meaningful activity, mastery is not easily gained. Almost all achievement includes an experience of stress, that is, tension, pressure or strain.[1] The impetus to grow, to learn, the stimulus of school, the inner drive of the child to explore can all be seen as stresses. They are pressures inching a system toward positive change. Stress, however, can reach a critical tension, no longer positive when pressure and demand for change temporarily overwhelm the individual's capacity to adapt. Dysfunction, physical, psychological or both, is the result.

Occupational therapy intervention with patients under stress is not new. Common sense acknowledges the extreme emotional stress of serious illness, the physical stress of pain, the environmental stress of the sterile, white hospital. The recent explosion of stress literature in the medical community, however, has created an awareness of "stress" as a potentially destructive force in itself, manifesting an array of physical and psychological illnesses including cancer,[2] arthritis,[3] and cardiac disease.[4] With this increase in information, occupational therapists are now able to more completely consider stress management a life skill, incorporating stress management activities into activities of daily living, exploring stress management as a component of independent living and competent role management. To begin this process, this article will review the components of stress, the stress cycle, intervention to manage stress, occupational therapy role and program models through case presentation.

STRESS—COMPONENTS AND RESPONSES

Stress may be viewed as a composite of the physical, emotional and environmental factors. By far the greatest physical stress encountered is pain. Physiologically, pain is a signal which informs us about potentially harmful stimuli. Eight of the most common pain syndromes treated in the medical setting represent the terrible scope of the pain experience. They are:

1. Vascular pain resulting from dilation of blood vessels in the periphery or the dura mater of the brain;
2. The muscle and joint pain of inflammatory processes or structural damage: including arthritis, bursitis, tendonitis, intervertebral disc disorders, low back syndrome and temporomandibular joint problems;
3. Causalgia, intense burning pain resulting from trauma to peripheral nerves;
4. Neuralgia, sudden, excruciating pain usually arising from the sensory neurons in the trigeminal nerve distribution of the facial region;
5. Terminal cancer pain generated by tissue destruction or obstruction of major organs;
6. Thalamic syndrome in CVA, the drastic lowering of pain threshold on the hemiparetic side of the body;
7. Phantom limb pain resulting from neuromas, scar formation, bone spurs or poorly understood descending pain messages arising from the brain;
8. And finally, post-surgical pain, especially in the abdominal region.[5-9]

Emotional pain is no less formidable. Like physical pain it varies greatly in intensity. It ranges from loss of reality contact, to grief, fear of an uncertain future, to material worries such as getting to the bathroom or paying the bills. Underlying both physical and emotional stress can be the pain of coping with a disorganized, unfamiliar or an extremely demanding environment. Intensive Care Units (ICU) exemplify such environmental stress with 24 hour light, noise, activity and bodily "invasion" of the patient. What is common to all faces of stress: physical, emotional, environmental and especially to combinations of these factors, is that they can elicit in a person the stress response.

The stress response is the result of behaviors learned early in life for coping with difficult and painful experiences. On the most primitive level, stress is perceived by the systems as a threat to its existence and leads to the flight or fight response. The body's regulating system then gives the order to increase metabolic rate in preparation to confront or escape threat. Physical manifestations of the flight or fight response include: increased heartbeat, a rise in blood pressure, rapid shallow breathing, release of adrenalin and other hormones, pupil dilation, tensing of skeletal muscles for movement, the constriction of blood flow to digestive organs and extremities, increased blood flow to the brain and major muscles, increased perspiration and release of stored sugar from the liver for energy.[10] If the body is not given relief from the biochemical changes that occur during fight or flight, a state of chronic stress is the result. Chronic stress or a prolonged state of threat causes damage to the body and potentially system deterioration and death. It is important to remember that emotional responses to stress can trigger the same or similar physical changes as fight/flight responses do in more life threatening situations. Hence, emotional stress becomes a cause of physical illness, pain and more emotional stress and the vicious cycle is established.

INTERVENTIONS

Medical science and psychiatry have a long history of response to stress related illness. Much of physical and psychological pain has been managed with an array of pharmacological agents such as analgesics, antispasmodics, sedatives, tranquilizers, narcotics or antipsychotics. In severe cases neurosurgical or abative procedures have been used. However, less drastic, non-invasion techniques are also available. Many of these are noted in Figure 1.

All of these non-invasive stress management techniques are used to induce a relaxation response. The relaxation response counteracts chronic stress by returning the body to its natural state of physical, emotional, and mental balance. This response is characterized by: decreased oxygen consumption, decreased respiratory rate, decreased heart rate, increase in alpha brainwave, decreased blood pressure, decreased muscle tension.[10] If the relaxation response can be elicited it becomes possible to break the chain of destructive physiological changes that occur in stress.

Occupational Therapy

Using the Kielhofner-Burke[11] model of human occupation one can consider that the occupational therapist's point of intervention for patients with stress related problems rests in the skill building or performance sub-system. The occupational therapist helps patients to develop skills upon which they can build habits of living consistent with their goals and the demands of the environment. Oc-

```
    I.  Distraction

        A.  Concentration
        B.  Listening
        C.  Breathing
        D.  Rhythm
        E.  Activities

   II.  Relaxation Techniques

        A.  Autogenics
        B.  Visualization
        C.  Guided Imagery
        D.  Desensitization
        E.  Progressive Relaxation
        F.  Meditation
        G.  Breathing

  III.  Cutaneous Stimulation

        A.  Vibration
        B.  Acupressure (Do-In, Shiatus and Jin-Shin-Do)
        C.  Eastern Movement Techniques
        D.  EMG Biofeedback
        E.  Contralateral Stimulation
        F.  TENS
        G.  Heat/Cold

   IV.  Adjunctive Stress Reduction Techniques

        A.  Time Management
        B.  Systematic Desensitization
        C.  Thought Stopping
        D.  Assertiveness Training
        E.  Rational Emotive Therapy
```

FIGURE 1

cupational therapy seeks, through the use of purposeful activity, to reverse vicious, and support benign cycles of adaptation.

The tools of the therapist are activity analysis and patient evaluation. The safe and effective use of stress management techniques in a therapeutic setting requires careful assessment of the patient's strengths and needs. Before choosing an activity a therapist needs to know the patient's status with regard to sensory, motor, cognitive, psychological and social functioning.[12] The activities themselves must be scrutinized to assess the demands they place on patient systems. Options for activity modification must be considered. With a goal of initiating a benign cycle of adaptation, occupational therapy treatment begins activity programming with a match between patient skill level and activity demand. For example, in using relaxation techniques, or mental activity with a patient who has a history of psychosis or poor ego boundaries, the therapist uses activities such as progressive relaxation or autogenics which heighten body awareness and attention to the present reality. Visualization and guided imagery, both non-reality based methods, would be avoided. Conversely, the patients with pain or severe somatic complaints may use more effectively the techniques which draw their attention away from physical sensation and the "offending" body part. Visualization, guided imagery and/or craft activities may later be varied and graded to expand the skill base in any deficit area affecting personal independence and life satisfaction. For example, the resting and emptying of the mind implied in meditation may be precisely the need of the colitis patient experiencing anxiety attacks. However, such a patient may lack the physical control and ability to concentrate required by such an activity. Starting with breathing and a rhythmic sport such as swimming may be an effective alternative in building tolerance for relaxation and control of anxiety. Learning new skills, and experiencing success will allow the system to become self-regulating, versatile and independent. An examination of specific program models and case studies will be used to demonstrate the application of these principles.

PROGRAM MODELS

Intensive Care

Requisites for admission to intensive care (ICU) at Stanford University Hospital include patient's need for invasive monitoring of vital systems, 12 hours/day nursing care, peritoneal dialysis or mechanical ventilation. Medical conditions that potentially create this demand are many, including adult respiratory distress syndrome, major surgery such as open heart or organ transplant, or vital system failure. In addition to experiencing an acute life threatening illness, the intensive care unit creates a challenge to patient adaptability. The ICU presents the patient with all of the four major components of the low stimulus environment.[13]

1. Sensory deprivation or lack of visual, auditory, tactile and kinesthetic input;
2. Perceptual deprivation or meaningless or unpatterned visual and auditory stimuli;
3. Immobilization: severe restriction of freedom of motion;
4. Social isolation: monotony and lack of social contacts.

The effects of such environments on people may include loss of motivation, impaired ability to concentrate, to maintain thought, to reason and problem solve; impaired visual perception processing and decreased dexterity.[14] Emotional states of anxiety, anger, guilt, shame or depression often parallel a sensory deprivation experience. The delusions and hallucination characteristic of patients in low stimulus environments may be a component of perceptual dysfunction. Zuckerman notes the system's effort to remain integrated by providing itself with internal stimuli to which it may respond in the event of environmental impoverishment.[14]

Another major stress of the ICU experience is that of ventilator weaning. The goal of mechanical ventilation at the onset of treatment is to stabilize the patient hemodynamically by adjusting the number of mandatory breaths per minute, percentage of oxygen received and the amount of pressure offered by the ventilator.[15] Once the patient's blood gases are stable, the goal is to slowly reduce mechanical intervention and oxygen support until the patient can breathe independently again. The process must be slow in order to allow the body to accommodate to fewer breaths and to lower oxygen concentration. The process is described by patients as physically tiring and emotionally stressful due to the resultant sensation of breathlessness or "air hunger". Since a fight or flight response during a period of air hunger would only increase oxygen demand and exacerbate shortness of breath, it is important to help the patient develop skills to cope to the rising sense of panic that breathlessness induces.

Awareness of the effects of low stimulus environment is most powerful when juxtaposed to the literature regarding the role of activity in coping with a stressful situation. Gal and Lazarus cite the importance of activity in enabling persons under stress to achieve a sense of mastery, and through this experience of personal effectiveness, to cope with even life-threatening situations more skillfully.[16] In viewing activity as a coping mechanism two major goals were noted: (1) activity directed toward dealing with the threat and (2) non-related activity performed in anticipation of stress. "Directed activity" in occupational therapy can be seen in tasks of daily living or crafts used specifically to increase strength, endurance or to enhance recovery. "Non-related" activity includes use of hobby, craft or relaxation exercises prior to an unpleasant procedure such as chemotherapy. It seems that depending on personality and context, distraction and/or direct effort to act upon stress can be helpful in enhancing a patient's sense of efficacy and ability to manage stress. The extreme inactivity imposed on the patient in the low stimulus environment of intensive care contributes further to vicious cycles of deprivation, disorientation and disengagement from life.

From this knowledge of the patient experience in ICU, the role of occupational therapy can be developed.

In general the therapist works:

1. To reduce the damaging effects of low stimulus environment through stimulation and environment enrichment.
2. To reduce stress of the ICU experience by empowering patients to participate in care and by adapting activity to meet medical restrictions and patient capability.
3. To assist patients to regain activity of daily living independence, including breathing, through participation in a ventilation weaning program.
4. To prevent rehabilitation complications when possible through splinting, positioning and adaptive devices.

The following case study illustrates occupational therapy programming used to reduce stress of one ICU patient.

M.T., a 58 year old female, was admitted to a Stanford Hospital ICU with the diagnosis of capillary leak syndrome, secondary to salmonella poisoning. Her past medical history was non-contributory with the exception of repeated history of sepsis of unknown etiology. Prior to hospitalization she lived with her husband and was independent in all aspects of self-care, working full-time as a secretary.

On day two of admission M.T. developed acute respiratory distress syndrome (ARDS), hypotension, anemia and angioedema. She was intubated and put on a respirator at an intermittant mandatory ventilation rate of six breaths/minute (IMV6). She had numerous invasive lines for monitoring hemodynamics and vital functions including (1) Swan-Gantz catheter, (2) right radial arterial line, (3) central venous pressure line, (4) subclavian line for transperenteral nutrition. Due to impending compartment syndrome bilateral fasiotomies of both lower extremities were performed.

The patient was alert and oriented at the time of the initial occupational therapy evaluation. She was unable to speak due to the endotracheal tube for ventilation and made little effort to communicate. She was at least passively cooperative and tolerated a physical assessment including tests of ROM, strength, sensation, motor function and activities of daily living. These tests revealed compromised strength and a need for moderate assistance for self-care activities of mobility, transfers and hygiene. M.T. was able to communicate with gestures and, with effort, was able to write. When she did write, her messages were one word demands expressing immediate urgent need such as "TURN", "WATER", or "STOP".

When asked questions in regard to her emotional status such as "How do you feel?" the patient always responded with a blank expression or a forced smile. She would then write "FINE". It seemed to both the therapist and nursing staff that M.T. was unable or unwilling to express fears, thoughts or needs in any greater depth. Nursing and physical therapy services observed that the patient required unusually high levels of support and encouragement to participate or to even cooperate in her care. During the next two encounters with M.T., the therapist focused on establishing rapport, encouraging M.T. to express her thoughts and concerns. Understanding more about M.T.'s perception of her experience seemed critical for setting goals and targeting treatment activities. During the interview process M.T. shared that prior to admission she loved to cook and to garden. She took great pride in her appearance and femininity. She felt embarrassed by her "sickly" appearance now and resented the fact that she had to use a bed pan. She was also afraid and somewhat resigned to the fact that she might die. She expressed anxiety about the ventilation and stated (in writing) that sometimes she felt that she was "going crazy".

After the first three visits by the therapist, the following problem list was established for this patient.

1. generalized weakness
2. moderate dependence in all activities of daily living
3. limited communication
4. ventilator dependence
5. anxiety, depression and fear, high risk disengagement from life, loss of motivation to live
6. sensory deprivation: feeling of being "crazy", boredom

A treatment program was established based on patient goals to begin to become more independent and less anxious. Specific patient concerns included: obtaining commode privileges and reducing feelings of panic. Responding to these needs was the first part of the full occupational therapy program.

For stress management, visualization and guided imagery relaxation techniques were introduced. The techniques were selected because of the patients strong need to at times escape the ICU, to focus attention toward health and away from her physical entrapment in bed, and because these techniques do not make high demands for concentration. Because of her strong ego boundaries, it was felt guided imagery would not be detrimental to M.T. Rather, mental activity to keep her connected with the things in life that she loved and her sense of self seemed vital to support her motivation to live. A progressive activities of daily living program was also established in conjunction with nursing service with the short term goal of allowing the patient to use a bedside commode rather than the bed pan. By removing what was, to the patient, a demeaning aspect of her care, she was able to exert some control of her environment. A sense of personal effectiveness boosted her sense of confidence in her recovery.

On day 15 of ICU admission, M.T. was ready to begin her ventilation weaning program. By this time M.T. was independent in the use of visualization tapes and was able to set, monitor and regulate her own stress management program for the difficult weaning process.

On day 25 of ICU admission, M.T. was extubated and breathing on her own. She was alert and oriented. Her self-care activities required supervision because she still required oxygen by nasal canula. She was transferred to a ward and 6 days later discharged home. At discharge she was independent in self-care skills. A 6-week follow-up revealed that she continued to find stress management activities to be a significant aspect of daily living.

Leukemia

The Compromised Host Unit (CHU) treats patients who because of serious blood disorder and immunosuppression require reverse isolation. The primary diagnosis of leukemia in patients seen on this unit include acute and chronic lymphocytic leukemia (ALL, CLL) and acute and chronic myelogenous leukemia (AML and CML). The prognosis of these diagnoses vary, ranging from approximately 4-6 months for types of AML to three years for ALL, CML and CLL.[17]

The principles of treatment on the CHU are outlined in protocols that vary from diagnosis to diagnosis. Drug toxicity is one complication common to all the varied forms of the chemotherapy regimes used to treat leukemias. This drug toxicity usually results in gastro-intestinal and central nervous system distress as well as bone marrow suppression and an increase in susceptibility to infection.

In addition to the physical distress of their illnesses, these patients are faced with the emotional issues relating to the death and dying process, the grief process, and accompanying feelings of fear, anger, guilt and lack of control. Because medical status mandates isolation, patients find themselves dealing with potentially devastating emotion issues in a solitary and confined low stimulus environment. Social and sensory deprivation and profound stress to a system already suffering for a physical and bio-chemical breakdown.

The following case study is used to demonstrate the importance of addressing the maladaptive stress response when treating a patient on the CHU.

C.S., a 40 year old male with a primary diagnosis of ALL was admitted to the Compromised Host Unit presenting with symptoms of a prolonged sore throat, stiff neck, splenomegaly and generalized fatigue. Blood tests revealed anemia and thrombocytopenia and bone marrow aspiration confirmed the diagnosis. Two days later a Hickman catheter was inserted and a chemotherapy regime began. An occupational therapy referral was written day 1 of admission.

Due to high risk of bleeding, patients generally set their own activity levels and do not receive any resistive testing from physical therapy or occupational therapy. Hence, the occupational therapy evaluation began with a functional check of physical status: pain, sensation, ROM, strength and coordination.

The evaluation also addressed cognition, emotional status, support systems, and ADL. Specific assessment tools used were the Life Stress Inventory,[10] the Interest Checklist,[18] and a Stress Symptoms Checklist.[10]

Test results revealed normal function on all physical parameters and independence in self-care. C.S. was cognitively intact and appeared knowledgeable and accepting of his diagnosis. He presented himself as extremely hopeful and positive. In fact, with hopes of successful induction of remission, he planned to be a candidate for a bone marrow transplant. C.S. had parents and two children ages 17 and 20 from a previous marriage living in the area. However, his wife of four years was his primary and consistent source of support during hospitalization. The patient has a wide range of interests. A policeman by profession, his avocation was flying his small airplane. He also enjoyed reading, artwork, and "all outdoor activities".

This patient identified chronic muscle tension, GI distress, and headaches to be his most common responses to stress. C.S. attributed the majority of the stress he experienced in his lifetime to his personal inability to express himself verbally or deal with his emotions. He even suspected that this deficit might have had something to do with the onset of leukemia.

While at the time of evaluation the patient was functional, a problem list was developed based on the seriousness of his diagnosis and the rapid change and fluctuation seen in patients physically and emotionally over the course of chemotherapy. This patient's problem list included:

1. high risk for deconditioning due to confinement and chemotherapy side effects
2. sensory deprivation/social isolation due to confinement with few visitors
3. high risk for maladaptive stress as physical discomfort of treatment emphasized to the patient the "fight for life" nature of the diagnosis
4. his expression of sense of losing control, feelings of fear over dependency on unpleasant procedures

From the beginning of this patient's hospital stay and involvement with occupational therapy, he was given the choice as to whether or not he wanted to receive and continue occupational therapy. This gave the patient some sense of control in a period and time when his medical status and the primary treatment seemed out of his control.

The patient opted for a physical therapy exercise program to help maintain strength and movement in lieu of an activity program. To manage the confined atmosphere and the stress of the hospital regime a stress management program was offered by occupational therapy. A comprehensive program was developed since no particular technique was contraindicated for this individual. The patient was trained in the stress response and the use of relaxation activities to counteract this maladaptive response. Beginning with simple breathing techniques, advancing to guided imagery and finally visualization, the patient at the end of the third week was able to independently use these techniques prior to receiving anticipated noxious procedures (i.e. x-rays, blood tests, negative test results). The patient reported that this made him feel an increased sense of control over his environment. Now he was able to internally self-regulate his emotional response to the internal/external and events over which he had no control.

This patient did not respond to the first or second induction of chemotherapy. With the third induction, the patient was sent into remission with extreme bone marrow suppression. Over this time, became progressively more nauseous, weaker and cachexic. Now the potential problems identified early in hospitalization became real and needed to be addressed more aggressively.

Confined to his bed C.S. was now forced to take a more passive role in his ADL. It seemed that all of his energy was expended going to and from the X-Ray Department, and receiving tests. The stress management techniques learned earlier in the patient's hospital stay when he had the energy and ability to concentrate were by this time fully learned skills, integrated into his repertoire of resources. It no longer took effort to perform these techniques enabling the patient to maintain a somewhat adaptive cycle going on the emotional level even while his body was actively engaged in a vicious cycle that eventually led to his death. Throughout his hospital stay, the patient incorporated these techniques into all phases of treatment. He would use the breathing techniques when working in physical therapy to reduce the pain he experienced with ROM and exercise.

Prior to performing an anxiety producing ADL (i.e. attempting to eat while suffering from extreme nausea) the patient would use visualization to imagine this experience as pleasurable. The patient stated this decreased the anxiety he felt when anticipating activity and in turn reduced the level of nausea he experienced. The patient reportedly used this technique to dissipate the severe pain that resulted from infection, conquer many sleepless nights and come to grips with his imminent death.

At intermittent points throughout this patient's eight and one-half month hospital stay, he would complain about his inability to express the grief and fear he experienced due to his disease process. As discovered in the initial evaluation, this patient found it difficult to identify, express or face his emotions. It was during this time that visualization coupled with art therapy proved a successful method to allow this patient to vent his feelings, gain insight and come to some acceptance of his death, dying and grief process. Often it was only by sharing this work with his wife, that he was able to communicate and express the many emotions he experienced during this disease process.

C.S. incorporated these techniques into his daily fight for life. During the last two weeks of his life, C.S.'s family became involved with the use of these techniques, coaching the patient through the guided imagery exercises when he became too weak to initiate them on his own.

At this crucial and vulnerable time, this technique provided the patient's family with a mechanism which allowed them to feel a sense of control. It also provided a platform to support and help their loved one in a time when even a modern medicine was unable to forestall death indefinitely.

Anorexia Nervosa

Anorexia Nervosa is a disorder seen primarily in young women. It is characterized by severe weight loss, distorted body image and fear of obesity.[19] Onset is usually in adolescence and the illness can continue for many years, even into middle age. The case presented here is of a young woman with anorexia hospitalized on the Comprehensive Medical Unit (CMU) at Stanford University Hospital.

The majority of patients with eating disorders admitted to this unit are in their early twenties to early thirties, with a history of one to ten years of eating difficulty and weight loss. The CMU is designed to deal with a variety of psychosomatic disorders including anorexia nervosa, bulimia and chronic pain. In the milieu nature of the unit "community" is enhanced by a multidisciplinary team approach using a multi-modal philosophy. The staff is made up of psychologists, psychiatrists, nurses, physical and occupational therapists, dieticians, physicians and a social worker. Elements of psychodynamic, behavioral, medical and pharmacological management are combined to offer the patient the broadest possible system approach for dealing with their problems.

The patient education in stress management and program implementation is shared by several team members—the occupational therapist, physical therapist, nurse and psychologist. The occupational therapist is responsible for introducing and orienting the patient to the principles of stress management. The patient is evaluated by the therapist using the Life Stress Inventory and Symptom Checklist, after which the correlations between the stressors and symptoms are discussed with the patient. A stress management technique suited to the patient's symptom complex is then recommended, and the patient is trained in its use on an individual and group basis.

The physical and psychosocial problems encountered in patients with anorexia nervosa (AN), are particularly well suited to intervention through stress management. The holistic model of stress management which emphasizes the mind-body connection and one's ability to tap into this network, is a natural resource for the person with anorexia whose major problem is disruption of the normal healthy mind-body gestalt. Within the global dysfunctional picture presented by the person with anorexia there are problematic subsystems that stress management can directly effect. The following areas are addressed by occupational therapy programming.

Anxiety: A common experience for persons with anorexia, anxiety is especially high at the time of admission to the hospital due to disturbed body functions, life threat,[20] fear of hospitalization and fear of change. However, activities learned early in treatment can later be applied to anxiety producing situations in daily life such as meal time.

Phobias: Many persons with anorexia suffer from food phobias, having taught themselves to be afraid of high calorie foods. Systematic desensitization in a functional setting can help the patient to decrease these fears and reintroduce a variety of foods to her diet. Thought stopping can also be useful with phobias, and in dealing with other obsessive thoughts which provoke anxiety.

Self Control: A pivotal issue for persons with anorexia is the need to exert control over self and environment. Many persons with anorexia complain that they have never been able to initiate or self-maintain an activity. It is always done to or for them. For them, self-starvation and excessive weight control is the first rewarding sense of control they have experienced. Therefore, one of the merits of stress management pointed out to the client is that it is a mechanism of self-regulation, something that one can turn on or off at will.

Body Image: One of the characteristic traits of persons with anorexia is the severe disturbance in body image that accompanies their need to lose weight and stay thin. As Bruch[19] explained, these ideas are self-imposed and the patient will deny anything that conflicts with her goal to lose weight, including hunger, weakness and normal body functions. Stress management techniques with a strong physical basis (progressive relaxation, autogenics and breathing) can facilitate normalization of body sensations that the anorectic has learned to "turn off". Some body sensations patients report that are "new" or "strange" during relaxation sessions are return of hunger, floating, tingling, warmth in the extremities, a sense of separateness and wholeness, feeling their breath entering and leaving their lungs, and sexual stirrings. The client is encouraged to allow these sensations to grow, and is reassured that they are "normal" feelings.

Positive body image can be reinforced by use of visualization with themes of health, beauty and self-esteem. Self-massage, in conjunction with visualization is used to desensitize the hypersensitive patient to touch and as a reality testing technique to help her distinguish between "fat" and other body structures such as bone, muscle and skin.

Creativity: For persons with anorexia the ability to create a response to a need within herself is often a new experience. It is a first step in learning to give herself what she needs, rather than relying on outside providers. There is also an element of risk in trying something new, for although she may have heard of many of the stress management techniques, the patient may never have been supported to try them herself. This small risk-taking reflects a willingness to be unique and original (different from family and friends), a characteristic of creativity.[21]

Other characteristics of the anorexia patient that support rapid learning of stress management techniques include her usually high intelligence, her strong need to control anxiety and her genuine commitment to doing well. Characteristics that may initially hinder the success of stress management are her fears of losing control and her inability to take responsibility of herself. The patient may complain that the physical effects of relaxation, especially the sensation of floating or lightheadedness, make her feel out of control. The patient can be told that these are normal psychological reactions and at first might feel strange or frightening, but with practice they become more comfortable and even pleasurable. Reassurance that she is in control and can bring herself out of deep relaxation at will is helpful. To engage the patient in taking responsibility for regaining her health, the program can be graded from short individual sessions to longer supervised ones and ultimately to independent use of techniques. Caution should be exercised in recommending techniques to a person with anorexia who may have other underlying psychiatric diagnosis such as depression or borderline personality. Visualization and meditation can accentuate the loose thinking or weak ego boundary of such a patient making the more physically based techniques more helpful.

Case Study

The following case study illustrates the use of a stress management program with one patient with anorexia nervosa.

A.F. is a 32 year old Caucasian female with a ten year history of anorexia nervosa. A secondary diagnosis of mitral valve prolapse was made during her hospitalization. When admitted to Stanford Hospital's CMU, she weighed 29.6K (55% of her normal body weight) and was suffering from life threatening cachexia, weakness and dehydration. Although ambulatory, her severe malnutrition and risk for sudden death promoted her physicians to order her on bedrest until she reached a stable weight. Psychologically, she was fearful, dependent and in denial of her poor physical condition. An occupational therapy referral was received the day of admission and evaluation was begun one week later due to the patient's activity restrictions. All areas of occupational performance were considered.

Behavioral Observations and Interview: A.F. presented herself as alert, oriented and pleasant. She was guarded in her responses and emotionally labile, becoming tearful at times. She admitted to feeling very anxious and upset about being restricted to bed, but stated she understood the medical necessity. Her appearance was extremely cachexic. Dressing and hygiene were independent if done in bed.

Bed mobility was functional. Transfers were not tested secondary to bedrest. Feeding was supervised intermittently to provide encouragement. She admitted to performing eating rituals that interfered with normal eating behavior.

Prior to admission A.F. enjoyed cooking for others and was independent in meal preparation and housekeeping. She stated her goals were to gain weight and learn more about proper nutrition and exercise. She also admitted to needing to change her thinking about her body and femininity. A.F. had many questions about the occupational therapy program and hesitated in committing herself. She was amenable to trying stress management training while in bed.

History Pertinent to Occupational Therapy: A.F. was a practicing professor in psychology at a major medical school. She lived alone but near her mother's home. Her only sibling, a brother, lived in the same city. A.F.'s father had been a physician and encouraged the family to maintain a healthy lifestyle, with an emphasis on weight control. Her mother was overprotective and rigid. A.F. left home to attend college across the country, the resulting separation from her family was very difficult. During her freshman year her father died and since that time she has complained of occasional periods of depression which have become more chronic over the years. She was in psychoanalysis for eight years but discontinued it when she decided it was ineffective. A.F. had never married, but dated frequently. She had a broad social network and support system through work and family. Her only prior hospitalization was a two week admission for weight gain under medical supervision. During the year prior to admission she had become increasingly concerned about her lack of energy, loss of interests and her inability to pursue meaningful social relationships.

Test Findings:

- — Functional strength test was within normal limits except for the complaint of difficulty climbing stairs.
- — Interest inventory revealed avocational interests that included reading, needlecrafts, theater, dancing and cooking.
- — Perceptual evaluation: a self portrait drawing showed distorted body image, A.F. reported seeing herself as fat and childlike.
- — Life Stress Inventory revealed major stresses including illness, sleeplessness, change in eating habits, change in work load, anxiety, lability, revision of personal habits and change in rec-

reation. Patient mentioned she also felt the loss of her father, and of a grandfather who had also died.

—The Symptoms Checklist revealed a constellation of sleep and gastrointestinal disturbances, chronic muscle tension and weakness.

The initial occupational therapy problem checklist included abnormal eating habits, low endurance, restricted activity level, anxiety, distorted body image, irrational thought processes, social isolation and difficulty making therapeutic alliance with the therapist.

The therapy plan was designed to normalize eating behaviors, increase endurance to allow a full activity program, decrease anxiety in general and specifically around eating, improve perception of body proportions and sensations, replace irrational self-talk with realistic self-perceptions, increase socialization and develop a therapeutic relationship. While many modalities were used in treatment of various problems, the role of stress management in the program will be the focus of this case analysis.

During the first week of therapy it was necessary to establish trust with A.F. and to introduce her to the basic elements of the program. Her anxiety concerning self-disclosure, compounded by fear of her weight gain, made this difficult. Relaxation training was begun to help diffuse the anxiety and help her feel safe with the therapist. Breathing techniques were presented first, as A.F. had identified this as the most acceptable activity to her. She could only perform minimal repetitions of each exercise due to abdominal weakness but she was able to move her center of breathing from her chest to her abdomen. After the first session A.F. reported less muscle tension in her neck, shoulders and stomach, increased warmth in her hands and feet and sexual arousal. She also noted a feeling of peacefulness and the need to be hugged or touched. A.F. was taught to use the breathing to "frame" mealtimes, thereby decreasing her "nervous stomach" and allowing her to eat more comfortably. She was very receptive to practicing on her own.

During the second week, individual training sessions helped A.F. to improve her skill and endurance in stress management activities. She reported more response in the form of muscle relaxation and lightheadedness. She independently used the technique to decrease anxiety at mealtimes. At this point, A.F. also began sharing more information regarding issues of control and fears of obesity.

In her third week of training she attended a relaxation group on the ward and was able to achieve deep relaxation in this setting. She shared her experience with group members and gave feedback on facilitating the relaxation response. Her weight gain allowed her to participate in ward activities and increase socialization. There was a noticeable decrease in her affective lability.

Weeks four and five emphasized diversification of techniques. A.F. tried autogenics with good results and began to use it regularly. She participated in a visualization exercise to identify childhood messages from her parents which contributed to her irrational ideas about femininity and independence. After identifying these ideas, A.F. practiced refuting these and developed positive self-affirmations to replace them. A.F. continued to attend the stress management group. Her eating improved, with fewer reports of tension and anxiety. She began to experience hunger more and no longer complained of being cold most of the time.

From the fifth to twelfth week A.F continued to practice breathing and autogenics independently. She tried progressive relaxation and found maximum benefit from it. She used techniques daily to decrease general tension, and to surround mealtimes and her family therapy sessions. During this period her weight steadily improved and she earned passes to leave the ward for shopping and socialization. She began trying fearful foods and cooked several meals herself. She requested and tried "thought stopping" to deal with her fearful self-talk about food. Her irrational ideas decreased and were replaced with goals and activities appropriate for her age and interests. She became increasingly aware of her bodily sensations and began differentiating hunger from anxiety ("nervous stomach").

During the last five weeks of her stay, A.F. was able to continue relaxation on her own and she discontinued attending the stress management group. She explored issues of femininity and sexuality and their relationship with her new source of control and direction. She began planning for going home.

Time management training was initiated to offer a structure for a balanced lifestyle at home, incorporating relaxation sessions on a regular basis. At discharge, A.F.'s behavior was social and age-appropriate. Her endurance and strength had increased to allow her full activity in self-care, work and leisure. She was able to meal plan and cook a balanced diet and had begun to enjoy eating in restaurants again. Although she continued to have occasional bouts of feeling fat, overall her body image was that of a healthy, attractive and sexual young woman. The anxiety and lability she originally exhibited were gone. She spoke hopefully of the future and the positive changes she had planned for her life.

CHRONIC PAIN

Pain patients comprise the second largest group of patients admitted to the Comprehensive Medical Unit (CMU). Their pain can be of two major types, physical (organic) or psychogenic. Patients experiencing either type have become increasingly incapacitated by their pain.

In such persons functional abilities have diminished and dependence upon family members has increased. The signs of physical pain that these patients exhibit include the commonly recognized characteristics of organic pain syndromes: cause by injury or disease, pain at injury or disease site, increased pain sensation with movement or palpation or decreased sensation with rest, analgesics or surgery. In its acute phase, physical pain will elicit the fight or flight response. As pain becomes chronic, that is 6 months or longer in duration, the reactive changes of acute stress diminish or disappear as the patient system makes varying degrees of adaptation.

Psychogenic pain is often vague or uncertain in origin. It may not have a precipitating event. The pain itself is indefinite, experienced throughout the body, often showing a discrepancy between the patient's perception of severity and his/her physical behavior in movement. The pain site may be ill-defined and change with position. It does not align itself with a referred site or neurologic dermatone. This pain can also be exacerbated by a wide variety of environmental stimuli, emotional stresses or mood changes.[22]

The following is a case study involving stress management treatment for a person suffering from psychogenic pain initially resulting from physical trauma.

G.R. was a 56 year old white female admitted to the CMU for chronic back pain and depression. Her primary roles as wife, homemaker, mother and grandmother had become severely limited, secondary to pain and her consequent need for bed rest. The apparent cause for this pain began with a fall at work in 1974 causing injury to the L4 and L5 discs, followed by major surgery and application of a full body cast. The pain continued resulting in four other back operations including a low anterior fusion of the lumbar vertebrae, nerve decompression, and joint dissection to decrease pain on the lower back nerves. None of these procedures brought relief. The patient sought help at a hospital-based pain clinic in San Francisco and, finally, came to Stanford Hospital with the intent of receiving further diagnosis and treatment through the Hospital's Pain Clinic. During hospitalization the treatment team addressed the biological, psychological and social issues compounding G.R.'s physical discomfort. Increasing the patient's ability to cope and function despite her physical pain was considered by the team in tandem with specific pain management.

An occupational therapy evaluation revealed deficits in the self-care, work and leisure components of G.R.'s daily life. She was independent in all self-care except when pain escalated to the point of her needing bed rest. At the time of evaluation minimal to moderate assistance was needed primarily in transferring from bed to bath, toilet, chair and automobile. Her endurance and sitting tolerance were extremely limited, such that the patient spent the majority of her day resting in bed to relieve pain. The work and leisure activities of the patient's day were also severely limited with G.R.'s husband assuming most of the homemaking tasks for which the patient had been responsible. Leisure pursuits now included sedentary activities that the patient could pursue in bed, such as reading, latch-hook rug making, television and visiting with friends. Previous interests had included entertaining, shopping, attending baseball games, church and theater. The occupational therapy problem list revealed pain, depression secondary to pain, decreased coping skills for dealing with stress and pain, decreased homemaking ability, decreased activity level, decreased socialization and leisure pursuits, decreased self-esteem secondary to the above.

The occupational therapy program for G.R. began with individual education in the nature of the stress cycle and the relationship of stressful events and the patient's own pain level. G.R.'s personal stress symptoms were identified using the Stress Symptom Check List. Individual relaxation training consisting of deep breathing, autogenics, and visualization were introduced to decrease somatization, to draw attention away from bodily discomfort and for use during pain flare-up. Time management training was used to balance energy expended in self-care, work and leisure activities with daily time for relaxation and rest to keep pain within functional limits. ADL activities were used to increase G.R.'s functional ability in self-care, work and leisure including meal planning and preparation while in the hospital. Instruction in and incorporation of energy conservation and work simplification into self-care and homemaking activities supplemented the ADL programming. Endurance was built by attendance at all occupational therapy group activities including programs of a graded sitting tolerance beginning with 15 minutes and progressing to a full length of stay (approximately 60 minutes). Finally, leisure activities involving others were used to increase social contact and to explore the environment outside the hospital.

At discharge, G.R. showed significant improvement in the performing of self-care, work and leisure components of daily life. Alleviation of problems noted by occupational therapy upon admission had continued and included a decrease in pain with the use of specific relaxation techniques and time management skills. As a result of relief from pain G.R. experienced a decrease in depression. She developed an awareness of pertinent physical and psychological stressors in her life and had learned and tested new coping skills in the form of stress management techniques. Functional improvements of special significance to G.R. included restoration of simple homemaking skills, increased activity level and greater tolerance for activities involving sitting and walking. This improvement freed her to expand social interaction and once again enjoy recreations such as attending baseball games and going shopping. Finally, the combined improvements in daily life, coupled with increased personal effectiveness and reduced pain served to boost G.R.'s self esteem and reported quality of life.

SUMMARY

This article has reviewed the phenomena of stress as an influence on health and quality of life. Stress that is not managed well can catapult the human system into a downward spiral of disease and disability. The learning, implementing and valuing of stress management offers the individual expanded options toward health. Using the Kielhofner-Burke model of human occupation as a frame of reference, one can view stress management as an element in each subsystem. It is a valued interest and goal at the volitional level. It is corporated into a pattern of living at the habituation level. It is built on skills developed at the performance level. To best promote a positive adaptation to life stresses, stress management activities should be incorporated into activities of daily living. The occupational therapist can play a key role in helping patients develop stress management skills, incorporate them into ADL and value them as their effect is noted. Activity analysis and patient evaluation guide the therapist in the selection of traditional (diversional and artistic) and non-traditional (relaxation training, mental activity) stress management modalities. The application of stress management programming is broad. As shown by the case studies presented in this article, it is a positive health behavior available and helpful to patients in a wide range of circumstances. Stress management can be a health enhancing part of daily life even when that life moves into intensive care.

REFERENCES

1. *Webster's New World Dictionary of the English Language.* Cleveland and New York, The World Publishing Co., 1957.
2. Siminton C and Matthews S: *Getting Well Again.* Los Angeles, Tarcher, 1978.
3. Selye H: *The Stress of Life.* McGraw-Hill Book Co., 1976.
4. Friedman M and Rosenman R: *Type A Behavior and Your Heart.* Fawcett Crest, 1974.
5. Beicher H: Pain in men wounded in battle. Ann Surg 123: 96, 1946.
6. Benoliel J and Crowley D: *The Patient in Pain: New Concepts.* American Cancer Society Professional Education Publication, 1974.
7. Drachman D: Pain of neurologic interest. *Am J Phys Med* 46: 544, 1967.
8. Johnson M: Pain: *The Subjective Symptom in Assessing Vital Functions Accurately.* Horsham, Pennsylvania, Nursing '81 Books, Intermed Communication Inc., 1981.
9. LeRoy R: Current Concepts in the Management of Chronic Pain. Miami, Florida, Symposia Specialists Medical Books, 1977.
10. Mason L: *Guide to Stress Reduction.* Peace Press, 1980.
11. Kielhofner G and Burke JP: A model of human occupational, Part I, Conceptual Framework and Content. *Am J Occup Ther* 34: 572-80, 1980.
12. Llorens L: Occupational Therapy Sequential Client Care Record Manual. RAMSCO Publishing Co., 1982.
13. Parent LH: Effects of low-stimulus environment on behavior. *Am J Occup Ther* 32: 19-25, 1978.
14. Zuckerman M: Hallucinations, Reported Sensations and Images. In *Sensory Deprivation: 15 Years of Research,* edited by JP Zubek. New York, Appleton-Century-Crofts, 1969.
15. Shapiro B Harrison R and Trout C: *Clinical Application of Respiratory Care.* Chicago, Year Book Medical Publishers, Inc., 1975.
16. Gal R and Lazarus R: The role of activity in anticipating and confronting stressful situations. *J Human Stress Dec:* 15, 1975.
17. Rubin P and Bakemeier R: editors for *Clinical Oncology for Medical Students and Physicians, University of Rochester School of Medicine and Dentistry.* Rochester, New York, American Cancer Society, 1978.
18. Matsutsuyu J: Interest Check List. *Am J Occ Ther* 22: 323-328, 1969.
19. Bruch H: Anorexia nervosa: therapy and theory. *Am J Psychiatry Dec:* 531-38, 1982.

20. Dally P and Gomez J: *Anorexia Nervosa.* London, Heinemen Medical Books Ltd., 1978.

21. Gottshalk LA: Psychoanalytic contributions to generation of creativity in children. *Psychiatry* Aug: 210-19, 1981.

22. Bond M: *Pain, Its Nature Analysis and Treatment.* New York, Churchill, Livingstone, 1979.

Occupational Therapy Intervention in Chronic Pain

Anne B. Blakeney, MSOT, OTR

ABSTRACT. Chronic pain is one of the most costly health problems encountered in our society today. The problems constituting the Chronic Pain Syndrome are typically composed of a complex array of sensory, perceptual, psychological, environmental and other factors which require the coordinated efforts of an interdisciplinary team. Occupational behavior provides a very useful frame of reference for the occupational therapist treating the chronic pain patient. This biopsychosocial approach focuses on well behaviors and functional role performance. This paper provides an overview of chronic pain and presents occupational therapy assessment and treatment strategies with chronic pain patients.

Pain is a universal human experience. Each of us has experienced pain at some point, whether it is a very sore throat which precedes an upper respiratory infection, or the sharp lower abdominal pain which may signal appendicitis. A complaint of pain, in one form or another, is reported to be the most common reason for a person to consult a health care professional.[1] Acute pain has the important biologic function of warning the individual that something is wrong and usually prompts him to seek medical counsel. It is also used by the physician as a diagnostic aid, as in the case of appendicitis.

In contrast to acute pain, chronic pain *never* has a biologic function. It may be defined as pain which (1) persists beyond the usual course of an acute disease; (2) persists beyond a reasonable time for an injury to heal; or (3) recurs at intervals for months or years.[2] Chronic pain becomes an end unto itself and the individual's life becomes significantly altered.

Anne B. Blakeney is Assistant Professor, Department of Medical Allied Health Professions, Division of Occupational Therapy, University of North Carolina at Chapel Hill, North Carolina.

CHRONIC PAIN SYNDROME

Chronic pain is one of the most costly health problems in our society today. According to Bonica,[2] data from numerous surveys indicates that over one-third of Americans have persistent or recurrent pain that requires medical therapy. Over 50 million persons are either partially or totally disabled by pain for periods ranging from a few days to weeks and months, and some are disabled permanently. Bonica[2] estimates that as a result of chronic pain, well over 700 million work days are lost, which, together with health care costs and payments for litigation, compensation, and quackery, totals nearly 60 billion dollars annually. In 1979, this figure equaled more than 10% of the U.S. national budget.

One must not confuse chronic nociception with the syndrome of chronic pain. For example, there are many sufferers of arthritis who have chronic nociception. However, in no way should they be included in the same category with the very depressed individuals who have chronic pain and an accompanying high incidence of medication dependency and disturbed social functioning.[1] Individuals with arthritis are often able to maintain functional occupational role performance with certain adaptations in their lifestyles. Chronic pain patients, however, are generally unable to do so.

Black[1] states that the Chronic Pain Syndrome is confirmed by "a significant alteration in the patient's lifestyle; his relations with other individuals; and a failure to show any progressive improvement while at the same time rarely becoming appreciably worse."[1 p. 210] The patient may suffer from multiple and intractable pain complaints, many of which do not correlate with existing physical problems or illnesses. An excessive preoccupation with these complaints is common on the part of the patient. Frequently family and friends as well appear to focus attention upon the patient's pain behaviors. Fear, depression, anxiety, and neuroticism may be present. The patient often cannot conceive of a future without pain and therefore has no realistic plans for the future, nor patience with any therapy requiring time or active participation on his part.[1]

SECONDARY PROBLEMS

The patient's concern over loss of income and work increases his anxiety. Disturbances in appetite and level of physical activity commonly follow. The use of narcotic and synthetic analgesics not only can cause depression but serve to magnify any depression already present. Sleep patterns become altered, either because of the pain or the continued use of drugs. Abnormal and unrestful sleep periods eventually result, causing a significant decrease in the feeling of well-being. This primary disturbance of the Circadian Rhythm leads to progressive physical and mental deterioration. In addition, confusion similar to organic brain syndrome may result from continued use of prescription and over-the-counter drugs.[1,2] In a significant number of patients pain tolerance decreases, possibly due in part to a chronic depletion of endorphins.[2]

Pain is an acceptable affliction in our society. It produces sympathy and support for the sufferer. Such environmental rewards in the form of attention by well-meaning friends and family often act to maintain the individual in the role of patient. Activities that might make the person feel worthwhile and promote function are often taken away by family and friends who end up unintentionally increasing the duration and severity of the chronic pain syndrome.[1,3]

CAUSES

Chronic pain may be caused by a variety of complex mechanisms. The scope of this paper does not permit discussion of each of these in detail. In general, acute pain which follows disease or injury produces autonomic reflex responses which normally decrease progressively and disappear in a short time. However, in some people these responses become excessive and constitute new sources of noxious stimulation.[1,2] Causalgia and reflex sympathetic dystrophies are examples. In others, environmental and psychological factors play the prominent role in the etiology and development of the chronic pain syndrome. To summarize, chronic pain may be caused by pathological processes, by prolonged dysfunction in the peripheral or central nervous system, or both, or it may be caused by operant mechanisms and psychopathology.[2]

The problems constituting the chronic pain syndrome are typically composed of a complex array of sensory, perceptual, psychological, psychosocial, environmental, and other factors which require the concerted and well-coordinated efforts of an interdisciplinary treatment team. Bonica[2] first developed, practiced, and wrote about this approach to complex pain problems over 30 years ago. However, he states, ". . . until recently the pattern of American medical practice was not conducive to such team efforts'' in the area of chronic pain management.[2, p.23]

In exploring the role which the occupational therapist may fill on such a team, it is useful to look first at the "Gate Theory" of pain control established and described by Melzack, Wall, and Casey[3-5] and at the model of treatment proposed by Wilbert Fordyce.[6,7]

THE GATE CONTROL THEORY

To understand the significance of the Gate Theory of pain control, it is useful to review briefly the history of medical practice and research in the area of pain. For 2 millenia, physicians accepted Aristotle's concept that pain resulted when an excess of vital heat caused an increase in the sensitivity of touch which was conveyed by the blood to the heart, and there experienced as pain.[8] Pain was thus viewed as a negative passion and a state of feeling opposite to pleasure. Despite the repeated attempts made by many anatomists, physiologists, scientists and philosophers who followed to prove that pain was a sensation felt in the brain, the Aristotelian concept prevailed.

The scientific study of pain did not begin in the modern sense until the 19th century when Majendie and Bell[8] demonstrated that the ventral roots of the spinal nerves are concerned exclusively with motor function and the dorsal roots with sensory function. In the years following this work, two opposing theories of pain developed. First, according to philosophers and psychologists, pain was purely an emotional experience. In opposition, scientists then viewed pain as purely a specific sensation with its own sensory apparatus independent of touch and the other senses.[8] By the middle of this century, the field of medicine had totally rejected the theory of the philosophers and the theory of specificity prevailed. Then Hardy and co-workers[8] reintroduced the duality theory. They proposed that pain has structural, functional, and perceptual energies. Though they felt that cutaneous pain thresholds were similar for everyone, they believed the reaction to pain was a complex physiologic process "influenced by cognitive functions and past experience, culture, and various psychologic factors."[8, p. 751]

In 1965, Melzack and Wall[5] introduced the Gate Control Model for Pain. As explained by Melzack and Dennis[9] this theory offers an alternative to the traditional specificity model of pain. It proposes the following:

Neural mechanisms in the dorsal horns of the spinal cord act like a gate which can increase or decrease the flow of nerve impulses from peripheral fibers to the spinal cord cells that project to the brain. Somatic input is, therefore, subjected to the modulating influence of the gate before it evokes pain perception and response. The theory suggests that large-fiber inputs tend to close the gate while smaller-fiber inputs generally open it, and that the gate is profoundly influenced by descending influences from the brain. It further proposes that sensory input is modulated at successive synapses throughout the projection from the spinal cord to the brain areas responsible for pain experience and response.[9, p. 203]

Though this theory is viewed as speculative and has been criticized, it is considered to be the most influential and important current theory of pain perception,[10] and it has stimulated a tremendous amount of research in the area of pain and pain control. It views pain perception and response as complex phenomena, "resulting from the interaction of sensory-discriminative, motivational-affective, and cognitive-evaluative components."[11, p. 81]

Thus, the Gate Control Theory may be helpful in explaining how diversion may decrease the intensity of pain. It proposes that a neural mechanism in the spinal cord acts like a "gate" to facilitate or inhibit the flow of nerve impulses from the periphery to the central nervous system. In addition, a central control mechanism is proposed which modulates pain perception and the responses produced by psychological factors or psychological control techniques.

Psychological factors may "mediate pain by altering individuals' appraisals of the threat, their ability to control the quality of noxious sensations, and their emotional arousal."[11, p. 81] Thus, pain may be abolished entirely, or at least the perception of the intensity of noxious stimulation may be reduced by psychological factors and control techniques.

This theory may provide a neurophysiological rationale which would support the concept of using purposeful activity with the chronic pain patient. Purposeful activity could increase the amount of sensory stimuli, particularly large-fiber input, going into the periphery and would alter the activity of the central control mechanism in modulating the perception of pain and the responses to any noxious stimulation. The cognitive, perceptual, and emotional factors which contribute to the central control mechanism would also be altered when one is engaged in purposeful activity.

TREATMENT

In considering medical management of chronic pain patients and the use of interdisciplinary teams, Fordyce offers a behavioral approach. Though this approach may differ from that which occupational therapists use in many settings, the contributions Fordyce makes in demonstrating the complexity of pain behavior should not be overlooked.

Fordyce[6] maintains that clinical pain tends to be viewed from the biomedical model, or disease model, only. While this model is helpful in understanding and treating acute pain, the persistence of problems beyond the healing efforts of the disease model indicates that another approach is needed. Fordyce proposes a treatment approach for chronic pain based upon a behavioral model. From a model conceptualized by Loeser,[6] he establishes the rationale for a behavioral approach based upon the following definitions:

> *Nociception* refers to actual stimuli impinging on peripheral nerve receptors (A-delta and C fibers).
> *Pain* refers to a sensory experience elicited by the perception of nociception. It is not this pain that the pain patient manifests, however. The sensation of pain activates higher nervous centers, leading to suffering.
> *Suffering* refers to negative affective responses generated by pain and by other situations, such as loss of a loved one, stress, anxiety, etc. Suffering in turn generates pain behavior.
> *Pain Behavior* refers to all forms of behavior generated by the individual, commonly understood to reflect the presence of nociception, including speech, facial expression, posture, seeking health care attention, taking medications, and refusing to work.[6, p. 235]

As one progresses through each step from nociception to pain behavior, new factors are introduced. The linkage between nociception and each succeeding element may diminish. Each element after nociception may occur for reasons entirely separate from the original nociception. It is pain behavior which constitutes our clinical observations about chronic pain. Many clinicians think they are dealing with nociception-pain, when in fact they are confronted almost exclusively with pain behavior.

Fordyce[6,7] maintains that behavior has significance in its own right; that it is not merely an extension of nociception, but that it is influenced by stimuli and reinforcement in the environment. Secondly, effectiveness of intervention is to be found in the ensuing behavior of the individual. Whatever the treatment, if the individual does not change his behavior, little has been accomplished. Thirdly, measuring the effectiveness of treatment is done not by verbal reports contributed by the patient or by subjective judgement, but rather by counting the frequencies of relevant events, or behaviors, which occur.

Fordyce[6,7] states that the pain behavior which begins in response to nociception may eventually occur totally, or in part, for other reasons. Specifically, it may occur because of reinforcing consequences provided in the environment. Therefore, pain behaviors may continue to occur over time in response to some underlying nociceptive stimulus, or, once established, in response to environmental reinforcement. In the latter case, the pain behaviors themselves function as operants in the individual's overall behavior patterns. Clinical experience indicates that some mixture of these two situations is common.[6]

Operant pain may evolve 3 ways: (1) through direct reinforcement of pain behavior (attention otherwise not received), (2) indirect reinforcement (avoidance of unpleasant events), and (3) punishment, or negative reinforcement, of well behavior.[6] For example, family members will admonish a patient from undertaking physical activity long after healing has occurred.

An individual with an acute illness is likely to resume well behaviors when recovery occurs. However, in chronic illness the reduction of symptoms does not lead automatically to the resumption of well behaviors. Disuse of certain behaviors may leave one only marginally capable of performing, just as disuse atrophy results in a lower level of muscle performance. Therefore, treatment must systematically attempt to identify and remediate deficits in the patient's well behavior patterns. Fordyce[6] states:

> Treatment must also provide opportunity for reengaging the patient into the life roles which constitute the well behavior repertoire. There must be systematic effort at reinstituting the vocational and avocational activities which keep people going in life . . . Reliance solely on a disease model concept of chronic illness and chronic pain leads one to ignore or underestimate the importance of these considerations.[6, p. 248]

OCCUPATIONAL THERAPY INTERVENTION

Occupational behavior provides a very useful frame of reference for an occupational therapist treating the chronic pain patient. Activity levels and functional status are evaluated in the areas of work, play, and self-care. The focus is on wellness. An individual's strengths are determined and treatment is begun by building upon established strengths. The goal is to increase well behaviors and functional activities in areas where role dysfunction is identified. Purposeful activity is used in intervention.

The Pain Clinic at The University of North Carolina at Chapel Hill (UNC) serves primarily an outpatient population and provides consultation services. Patients are referred from across the state by their local physicians and are evaluated by neurosurgery, neurology, psychiatry, anesthesiology, psychology, physical and occupational therapy, and dentistry. In the occupational therapy consultation, the occupational behavior frame of reference is used to guide assessment procedures and treatment considerations. Work and play histories are taken; daily activity levels are assessed; and current vocational and avocational interests and skills are reviewed. The individual's future plans, personal concept of health and wellness and expectations of the UNC Pain Team are determined. Recommendations are then made to bring into balance levels of activity and inactivity and the areas of work and play. In addition, patient education regarding individual responsibility for health care is often recommended.

CASE VIGNETTE

The following case vignette serves to illustrate the use of this approach. Mrs. T. was a 56 year old married woman and mother of five grown children. She resided in a rural community. Her chief complaint was oral-facial pain of 8-9 years duration and a fear of losing her teeth, despite reassurances from dentists that this was unlikely. Various medications had proven useless in controlling her pain.

Her work history revealed consistent work patterns in a variety of occupations (seamstress; shoe-construction; cook; etc.) since age 19. Recently, her pain had caused some absences from work. Her leisure interests included dancing, which she would have enjoyed more often, gardening, and tending to her house plants. Three years ago, she had overcome a life-long fear of water and taught herself to float in her daughter's pool. In the future, she envisioned herself continuing to work, and also she hoped to have at least one opportunity to travel.

Her play history indicated a lack of play skills. At 8 years of age, she had assumed all homemaking activities for a family of eight. Her mother was incapacitated with back pain ("lumbago"), and, as the eldest daughter, Mrs. T. had been assigned these homemaking responsibilities. She was not allowed to finish school which she regretted. She stated her mother had consistently told her she "did not need an education to become a wife."

At 16 she married a man twice her age and had three children in the following three years. Any independent behavior which she exhibited angered him and he often became abusive as a result. She divorced him at age 19 and remarried shortly thereafter and had two more children.

She continued to assume a dependent role in this relationship and deferred major decisions to her husband, as she had done in her first marriage and previously, with her parents. As a result, she had failed to develop a real sense of autonomy or any sense of independence and self-worth as a separate individual.

She now relied primarily on her youngest son and a daughter-in-law for social and emotional support. She felt a lack of understanding and emotional support from her husband, though she was unable to communicate this to him. She was at risk for losing support from the son, who was getting ready to leave for college, and the daughter-in-law, who had recently separated from her husband. Mrs. T. identified both of these situations as stressful for her. In addition, she felt her job in a school cafeteria was stressful. She sensed a lack of communication and support from co-workers. She stated feeling "helpless and lonely" when her pain was severe, and this was a source of stress.

She had no form of regular exercise and she was overweight. She described her life as "all work and no play" and indicated a desire to "have more fun."

Mrs. T. was assessed as having been unable to develop autonomy and the skills necessary for independent decision making and problem solving. These skills begin to develop in adolescence, at which time she was forced to continue in a dependent role with her first husband. She transferred this role behavior into her second marriage, and the subculture in which she lived tended to support this role for married women.

In her childhood she had not been allowed to play very often and, therefore, she had developed few skills for self-entertainment. In addition, her socialization skills appeared to be poorly developed, as she was unable to initiate requests for needed assistance at home or at work or to engage easily in casual conversations. Consequently, she felt lonely much of the time.

Two major strengths were identified: maintaining her worker role and her ability to overcome her fear of water and learning to float. This was used as a starting point on which to build a plan for intervention. It was suggested that she be encouraged to enroll in adult swimming classes in her community. This would serve several purposes: (1) it would continue the development of a leisure activity which she had already initiated; (2) it would provide her with physical activity and help control her weight, which she hoped to be able to do; (3) it would provide her with a sense of individual mastery and confidence which she needed; and (4) it would give her a new peer group with whom she could interact and possibly begin to develop better social skills.

It was also recommended that personal counseling be considered for the purposes of helping her gain a perspective on her accomplishments and encouraging her to become more assertive in seeking out and planning pleasurable leisure activities in order to bring her life more into balance. In addition, she needed to develop better communication skills so that she could ask for help and seek support from those around her.

The medical team's evaluation of this patient revealed no known etiology for her oral-facial pain. There were no significant factors obtained in her history which marked the onset of pain. When frustrated by a sense of loneliness and isolation, her pain problem appeared to emerge. She had perceived sympathy and support only at those times from her husband and most other family members.

Team members theorized that her pain behavior may have indicated a pattern of "learned helplessness" from early childhood, when she had been exposed to the support her mother received from having had back pain. This served as a role model for her throughout her life.

The physician acknowledged for the patient that the team knew and accepted the fact that she was suffering. Because no physical reason could be determined for the pain, a strategy for managing her life around it became the focus of treatment. The occupational therapy recommendations were incorporated as an integral part of the total plan for this patient. Learning positive approaches for seeking support when stressed and taking initiative for developing pleasurable activities became primary goals for this individual.

A limitation of the consultation setting is the lack of opportunity to guide a patient through the activities suggested for skill development and to monitor progress. As there was no occupational therapist available in this patient's community to carry out treatment recommendations, the development of social skills became a part of the goals for the counseling referral. Her local physician received a copy of the team's report as well. He was encouraged to monitor her progress and to provide positive support for her well behaviors. The recommendation to enroll in swimming classes was given to the patient to carry out independently, with her husband, son, and physician being advised to encourage and support her to do so.

CONCLUSION

Chronic pain is a complex phenomenon which affects many people in our society today. It is one of the most costly and frustrating problems which physicians encounter in clinical practice.

Melzack and Wall's multicomponent Gate Control Theory indicates pain is not a function of any one particular body system. Rather, the entire person is involved in the pain experience. Therefore, treating patients exclusively with surgery, anesthetic block, or other measures designed to block pain pathways may account for some of the frustration and failure in treating this complex problem.

Fordyce's behavior approach, though not indicated for all chronic pain sufferers, does offer a model for treatment which is compatable with the occupational therapist's assessment of occupational role performance. Occupational behavior provides a frame of reference for the therapist to follow in completing a comprehensive assessment and plan for intervention.

REFERENCES

1. Black R: The clinical syndrome of chronic pain. In *Pain, Discomfort, and Humanitarian Care,* Ng and Bonica, (eds) New York: Elsevier/North-Holland, 1980
2. Bonica J: Pain research and therapy: past and current status and future needs. In *Pain, Discomfort, and Humanitarian Care,* Ng and Bonica, (eds), New York: Elsevier/North-Holland, 1980

3. Melzack R, Wall PD: Pain mechanisms: a new theory. *Science,* 50:971-979, 1965

4. Wall P: The gate control theory of pain mechanisms: a reexamination and re-statement. *Brain,* 101:1-18, March, 1978

5. Melzack R, Casey KL: Sensory, motivational and central control determinants of pain: a new conceptual model. *The Skin Senses,* D. Kenshalo, (ed), Springfield, IL: Charles C. Thompson, 1968

6. Fordyce W: A behavioral perspective on chronic pain. In *Pain, Discomfort, and Humanitarian Care,* Ng and Bonica, (eds) New York: Elsevier/North-Holland, 1980

7. Fordyce W: *Behavioral Methods for Control of Chronic Pain and Illness,* St. Louis: C.V. Mosby Co., 1976

8. Bonica J: Neurophysiologic and pathologic aspects of acute and chronic pain. *Arch Surg* 112: 750-761, 1977

9. Melzack R, Dennis SG: Neurophysiological foundations of pain. In R.A. Sternbach (ed), *The Psychology of Pain,* New York: Raven Press, 1978

10. Weisenberg M: Pain and pain control. *Psychol Bull,* 84: 1008-1044, 1977

11. Turk D, Michenbaum D, Genest M: *Pain and Behavioral Medicine,* New York: The Guilford Press, 1983

Perspectives on the Pain of the Hospice Patient: The Roles of the Occupational Therapist and Physician

Kent Nelson Tigges, MS, OTR
Lawrence Mark Sherman, MD
Frances S. Sherwin, MA

ABSTRACT. Beyond the physical disfigurement and emotional ravages of advanced malignancy, it is the pain of cancer that is most dreaded. Severe biological pain is experienced by fewer than half of patients dying from cancer. Hospice physicians have the expertise to control the pain of those cancer patients who do experience it. The cancer patient may experience other forms of pain that can be equally devastating: pain of isolation, pain of abandonment, and pain of loss of role. It is important for the occupational therapist working in a hospice setting to understand all aspects of pain management, and be competent to deal with the pain of loss of role. This article addresses the physician's role in pain management and the occupational therapy treatment strategies which can improve the quality of life and perception of pain for the hospice patient.

Through presentation of case studies, the authors illustrate applications of occupational therapy assessments and interventions in respect to two hospice patients. The occupational therapy treatment strategies effected an improvement in the quality of life for these patients and consequently their perception of pain of loss of role. Occupational therapists, as part of the hospice team, play an important

Kent Nelson Tigges is Associate Professor and Associate Chairman of Occupational Therapy, School of Health Related Professions, State University of New York at Buffalo. He has studied and worked in Hospices in England and Scotland and is the resident consultant for Hospice Buffalo, Inc.

Lawrence Mark Sherman is the physician in charge of home care for Hospice Buffalo, Inc. He is a Board Certified General Surgeon, with an academic appointment of Clinical Instructor in the Department of Surgery, at the State University of New York at Buffalo, School of Medicine.

Frances S. Sherwin is assistant to the Dean, School of Health Related Professions, State University of New York at Buffalo. She has had extensive experience as a medical writer and editor.

55

part in giving patients an opportunity to live out their lives in as dignified and purposeful a manner as their disease permits.

It is not an unusual human assumption that life will be indefinitely healthy, happy, safe, secure, comfortable, and productive. It is also not unusual to assume that critical or disabling illness happens to others. The disclosure of a diagnosis of cancer, particularly advanced metastatic malignancy, can only be traumatic. The images that such a diagnosis conjures up are of unbearable physical and mental pain, deterioration, disfigurement, and death. Unlike the pain of benign disease, which signals a pathological process that a skilled physician may have the knowledge to cure, the pain of terminal cancer serves no useful purpose. It only reminds the patient of a grim prognosis.

The traditional goal of medicine is to cure the patient. Physicians treating patients with cancer hope to cure them of their disease or, failing that, hope to provide significant prolongation of life. Traditional medicine has set an exemplary record in providing cure for the vast majority of patients. However, for patients with advanced malignancy, traditional medical methods are inappropriate. The pain of the patient with extensive metastatic malignancy is caused by an insuperable source. It is constant, ranging in intensity from dull to severe. Therefore, it seems most appropriate to direct medical attention to eradicate the symptom itself. This is the hospice approach to pain control.

The traditional goal of occupational therapy in an acute hospital or rehabilitation center is to remediate the pathological problems interfering with occupational roles, or failing that, to focus on compensatory methods to assist the patient in maximizing his potential for a long and productive life. In the hospice setting, the goal of occupational therapy focuses on reducing the pain of loss of role by maximizing the patient's potential to regain as many former roles as possible within the context of a very short future.

BIOLOGICAL PAIN

Pain is a multifaceted phenomenon. Many different factors cause great variation in a patient's perception of pain. The perception of biological pain varies greatly among individuals. Pain stimuli may differ because of the concentration of injured pain-sensing nerves.

The same stimulus may affect different numbers of nerves in different subjects. Because concentrations of nerve fibers differ throughout the body, noxious stimuli are perceived differently. The degree to which the individual is distracted by other stimuli, as well as social, environmental, and cultural factors will modify both the perception of, and response to, painful stimuli. Feelings of anxiety, depression, and loneliness heighten pain perception, just as pain increases these emotions. Nonetheless, it is possible to categorize pain qualitatively into three types: mild, moderate, and severe. These categories are important in pain management, a central concern of hospice.

MANAGEMENT OF BIOLOGICAL PAIN

A practical plan of pain management in the hospice setting has evolved. A patient with pain from advanced cancer is studied to determine the source of his complaints as well as any environmental and emotional factors which may heighten his pain response. If the pain can be treated effectively at its source, such as by administering radiation to an enlarging mass or by immobilizing an unstable bone fracture, this will be the first step. All too often, however, the pain cannot be treated so easily and the physician is forced to resort to pharmacologic control. Appropriate medication depends on the severity of the pain. Mild pain is best treated by a class of drugs known as the nonsteroidal anti-inflammatories (NSAI), of which aspirin is the best known. Moderate pain requires an NSAI plus a mild narcotic, such as codeine. Severe pain requires appropriately strong narcotics, with or without an NSAI adjunct. It is only after the patient's pain is under some reasonable control that his emotional factors can be dealt with effectively.

The pain of cancer is constant. Therefore the analgesic control must be maintained on a constant basis. Pain from advanced cancer is controlled only by medication given around-the-clock, as opposed to medication on a PRN basis. It is well established that the dosage of medication given to maintain pain below the threshold of consciousness is not as high as that required once pain is perceived. Thus, many of the side effects of potent narcotics may be avoided or reduced considerably on an around-the-clock regimen at sufficient dosage.

The use of narcotics in the treatment of pain from advanced

malignancy is poorly understood by lay people as well as by many in the medical community. One concern is that the patient will develop addiction. Even if addiction were to occur, the hospice staff would dismiss that fear as unreasonable. In a patient with a short life expectancy, addiction to narcotics should be neither a social nor medical anathema. However, when narcotics are given appropriately (i.e., on an around-the-clock basis and at doses high enough only to relieve pain), addiction does not occur. If the dosages of narcotics are followed over time in a given individual, a stepladder increase as might be expected in an addict does not develop. Instead long plateaus are followed by decrements if the disease is responding to treatment or increments if progression has occurred. There are several explanations for the fact that cancer patients are not likely to become addicted. It may be that dosages of narcotics given are too small to produce a "high." Also, most cancer patients wish not to be so ill that they require narcotics, and therefore psychologic addiction rarely occurs. Likewise, the properties of narcotic analgesics are such that there is no point at which no more can be given. Dosages raised in a rational fashion can be increased indefinitely to the level required for analgesia in any given patient.

Another concern of patients is that they will become oversedated, "snowed" by the drugs. The fear is not unreasonable; all too often, this has been how narcotics have been used. But when appropriate pain relieving doses of narcotics are given on an around-the-clock basis, oversedation rarely occurs. After the initial forty-eight hours of drug use, narcosis should have disappeared entirely unless the dose employed is much too high. Patients on maintenance narcotics are able to work, drive, and behave in general in as normal an environment as their underlying disease allows.

PAIN OF ISOLATION

In addition to physical pain, people who are dying frequently experience the pain of isolation. Members of the health care team actually withdraw from the dying patient. They spend less time in the patient's room; examinations and assessments become more cursory, and physical contact is minimized. The terminally ill cancer patient is not brought to the occupational therapy department because he is too "sick and weak," and "other patients would be upset by his presence." The attitude tends to be that since occupational therapists are in the business of rehabilitation and making patients better, they cannot have a patient in their clinic who is not going to live. As the medical team abandons the terminally ill patient, so do family and friends, who visit less often and cut short their visits. Family and friends, also devastated by the diagnosis, fear mentioning the problem or the prognosis. Conversations are contrived, the reality of the situation is avoided, and gradually isolation occurs. As the patient becomes more critical, vigils are kept in silence.

PAIN OF ABANDONMENT

The pain of abandonment occurs when the professional team and family stop caring for the patient as a human being. Abandonment typically begins the day that the patient's diagnosis is known, and it generally begins with a lie. Either the doctor, the family, or both, feeling guilty or inadequate, are unable to confront the patient in respect to his impending death. No one wants to be the bearer of bad news, so to "protect" the patient they lie. Lies are rationalized because they wish to spare the patient any further pain. The patient who is told he has terminal cancer may "go to pieces," give up, and die sooner, and painful feelings and emotions may be avoided by pretending the situation is better than it is. The patient is dealt with at a "clinical" level, which is safer. Such approaches, although well intentioned, do a disservice to the patient because he will eventually discover the nature of the illness and the prognosis. He may respond to the deception with anger, severing bonds with the conspirators or, fearing abandonment, he may become a co-conspirator and pretend not to know the diagnosis. Such pretenses lead to artificial and strained communication and ultimately to no communication.

THE HOSPICE PHILOSOPHY

The hospice philosophy is that it is vital that the health team and family members convey honestly and compassionately their personal and emotional commitment to the patient. Because health care providers have been trained to save and rehabilitate lives, this task requires an entirely new perspective. Although the life cannot be saved, the final days, weeks, or months of life can be fulfilling. The health care team will continue to care for the patient, will continue to maximize the patients' potential, and will, under no circumstances, abandon the patient.

Diagnostic and prognostic honesty is necessary to minimize or eliminate the pain of isolation and abandonment. In fact, diagnostic honesty is one of the basic tenets of hospice philosophy. The assumption of hospice is that cancer patients have not only the right but the need to make decisions about their lives which cannot be made without sufficient information about their illness and its outcome. On admission, a Hospice Buffalo staff member makes the hospice position on diagnostic honesty clear to the family and primary caregiver. In the majority of cases, families are relieved by their honesty and openness. Some families will say that the patient does not know he has cancer, and family members have agreed not to tell. Hospice staff explain that they will not lie to the patient. However, there are many ways to tell a terminally ill patient he has cancer and is going to die. Sensitive and caring hospice staff leave the doors open so the patient feels safe, feels free to ask questions, and knows that he will be given honest answers and will not be abandoned whatever the prognosis. Hospice staff is prepared and expects to talk with the patient about his impending death. When the patient knows the truth, he can discuss plans realistically, he can consider options, and the energies he and others once used to camouflage the truth can be directed toward fulfilling realistic needs. The absence of a cure does not preclude relief of pain and other symptoms or possibility of a decent quality of life.

PAIN OF LOSS OF ROLE:
THE ROLE OF OCCUPATIONAL THERAPY

Once the physical concerns of the patient are under good medical management, his attention turns to the realities of everyday life. Typically, patients feel they no longer have a purpose in life. They experience the pain of loss of role. The following statement is a poignant reflection of these feelings.

> It was Sunday last. My husband, three children and I went to church. As I knelt I looked around and thought of all those who had prayed here over the centuries and who had gone before me. It was important for me to be there just one more time for

the next day I had to tell my family that although my operation was successful, the results were not, and that I had less than a year to live. I thanked God that my children were old enough to be reasonably independent. As I looked at them the pain began to grow—not to be there for the last high school graduation; I supposed someone would be there to make the tea and cakes but, you see, I have always been there to do it.

I looked around at all the other people. They looked so healthy and normal. It was then that I began to feel another kind of pain. I felt resentment that they would go home that day and laugh and enjoy life. For me now there would only be superficial laughter. Moreover, I felt the pain of losing my ability to be a friend. I was always so active and doing things for people. What would happen when I told them? Would they abandon me? Would they pity me—because I couldn't bear it if they would. I guess my greatest pain would occur when I would no longer be able to be the mother and wife I once was. My heart ached at the thought that I would slowly, and God help me to gradually and gracefully, have to rely more and more on my family and friends to do the jobs and tasks I once did. How could I bear the pain of becoming dependent?

Anonymous
St. Lukes Hospice,
Sheffield, England, July 1983

Panic can ensue, time is running out, health is fading, I am dependent, I am helpless and useless. It is during this period in the patient's illness that the occupational therapist can contribute most to minimize the pain of the terminally ill cancer patient. The therapist approaching practice from an occupational behavior perspective can diminish the pain the patient is experiencing. The occupational behaviorist* believes that quality of life extends substantially beyond the state of mere survival. Quality of life rests with internalized feelings of positive self esteem. By making a contribution people gain respect for themselves and the admiration of others.[1, p. 4] This respect and admiration leads to feelings of worth and positive self esteem—

---

*The term occupational behaviorist (Tigges) refers to an occupational therapist who is a strict adherent of the occupational behavior paradigm.

thus competency is realized and a purpose for living is recognized. The occupational therapist can assist the terminally ill person, who feels he has no reason to live, to realize potential through examining and supporting strategies for achievement in self care, work, and leisure.

THE OCCUPATIONAL THERAPY ASSESSMENTS

The person with terminal cancer is especially vulnerable during the assessment process. Recounting one's occupational history can evoke recollections of previous success, happiness, and independence, which are painful in light of current problems. If sensitively handled, the occupational therapist can facilitate the recollections of the past in such a manner as to build positive perspectives for future achievements.

Three of Reilly's specifications of the occupational behavior paradigm are significant for the attainment of quality of life for the terminally ill. First, patients must be given the opportunity for natural and legitimate decision making in regard to their medical care and how they choose to live their lives; second, patients must be permitted "normal living experiences performed at natural times"; and third, patients must be permitted a balanced existence: activities should be distributed among self-care, work, and play.[2, p. 63-4]

To implement these specifications, the occupational therapist carries out a three-stage assessment. The first stage assessment is the occupational history (Tigges unpublished) which provides a perspective on the patient's occupational roles, how his occupational choices were made, what position the person played within these occupational roles (i.e., independent, interdependent, dependent), which roles were regarded as essential, obligatory, preferred, enjoyable, and if a sense of mastery was achieved and recognized. In the context of occupational roles the therapist looks at generic roles throughout the patient's life; i.e., as an employed person, spouse, parent, grandparent, student. What a patient accomplished or failed to accomplish in the past has a direct impact on how he adapts and performs at the present and how he will cope and perform in the future.

The second stage assessment is temporal adaptation. The temporal assessment (Tigges unpublished) produces information on attitude towards time, time perspective and time allocation on a daily basis. Temporal adaptation queries reveal how the patient either controls time or lets time control him. More important, these questions provide invaluable information on how each patient views his past, present, and future within the time he had and the time he has left. Time can be the most coveted or feared aspect of life. The perception of time can be the single most important factor in achieving quality of life. It governs how and where the patient sees himself within the context of impending death. There is not a single individual who does not look forward to, and plan for, the future. Plans and hopes for the future are tied to time; "when I retire," "five years from now," "when I graduate" are the words used to express plans and hopes. When a catastrophic illness such as advanced cancer terminates the reality of a future, it is not uncommon to see people give up wanting to live another day. Daily achievements are meaningful only as they relate to some future plan or expectation. By assessing a patient's perspective on time, it is possible to alter and reconstruct his belief in a seeming paradox—that, in fact, there can be "hope without a future—a future without time."[3]

The third stage assessment is physical. The physical capacity of the patient involves assessment of muscle strength, joint mobility, coordination, endurance, balance, ambulation and sensory motor integration. How the patient and therapist set goals and what expectations can be realistically achieved are determined. Assessment is constant and ongoing. In acute care, and hospice is considered acute care, assessment and treatment planning must be accomplished expeditiously. The three-stage occupational therapy assessment can be accomplished on the initial visit to the patient, and the treatment program must be initiated immediately. To illustrate the applications of these specifications and assessments to occupational therapy interventions, the following case studies are presented.

CASE STUDY 1

In January of 1983, John, age 66, was diagnosed as having a jugular blastoma and a life expectancy of six weeks. Upon admission to hospice home care his wife was "appointed" as the primary care giver. Although John's biological pain and symptoms were controlled within 72 hours, he demonstrated a passive aggressive attitude. His relationship with his wife, which previously had been one of warm companionship, became stressed and confrontational. He refused to take his medication as prescribed.

The occupational therapy assessments revealed that John was born in a small rural community, the eldest son of seven siblings. He began to work at the age of 10 years on a neighboring farm. Following graduation from the eighth grade until he retired at 65, he held various jobs as a skilled laborer from which he received significant intrinsic gratification. He built his own home, was the sole breadwinner, was the father of two sons and a daughter, and was the central, stabilizing force in his family and the major decision maker. He lived through the Great Depression and knew about moderation, commitment, hard work, and responsibility.

John had always been in control of his life and in charge of his family. He expressed resentment that his wife had been arbitrarily made "head of the family." He resented that the family leadership role had been taken away without consulting him. He was painfully aware that as a result of his cancer, significant weight loss, and resulting physical weakness, he was incapable of carrying out all his previous roles. "Maybe I'm only half the man I once was, but I can still think. My judgment is good. Just because my body is shot doesn't mean I am completely useless."

Apart from being denied a role as head of the family, and decision-maker, he was angry that his wife and other family members were deciding what he should and could do with his life, what he should eat, and when he should rest. He disliked their decision that it would be best if he did not spend much time in his basement workshop for fear he would become weak and his wife would have difficulty getting him upstairs to his bedroom. In spite of the fact that he had been included in some of the conversations with the team and his wife, he told the occupational therapist that he felt like excess baggage. He was never the absolute center of attention and decision. "After all it is my life they are planning. None of their suggestions represent the way I want to spend the rest of my life."

The occupational therapist and John altered decision-making strategies. John was once again in the position of control as he had been for 50 years. By assisting John and his wife to return to their former, customary roles, their strained relationship was replaced by loving concern for each other. John set the priorities as to what he wanted to do each day. He wished to spend most of his day at his workbench so he could finish several very important projects. Once John's wife understood the importance of his being at his workbench and how to cope if he became too weak to climb the stairs, her anxiety dissipated. Thereafter, she encouraged him to work, which he did until two days before he died. The occupational therapist was able to help John acknowledge that his future consisted of passing on his skills and abilities to those he cared about. Those he left behind would always remember him because of what they learned from him. He taught his wife to manage the family's financial affairs, his sons to maintain their homes, and his grandson to shoot pool. This was his legacy.

CASE STUDY 2

Bill, a 29-year-old husband and father of an 18 month old son, was diagnosed as having pontine glioma. Following exploratory surgery and eight weeks in a hospital, he was admitted to hospice home care. Upon admission he was bedridden with left hemiparesis. Due to a 50-pound weight loss and significant muscle wasting, Bill was unable to bathe or dress himself. With the exception of standing and walking ten steps with maximum assistance, he was physically incapacitated. His physical care was provided by his wife. The initial hospice assessment showed that Bill was physically comfortable and extremely happy to be home with his family. He expressed no particular needs.

The occupational therapy assessment revealed that Bill had a B.A. degree in mathematics, and prior to his illness he had been a senior computer operator in a large international firm. Because Bill was a very retiring person, it took significant probing to reveal his needs and goals. He characterized himself as a quiet, shy person. "I was never outgoing, never very good at expressing myself."

Bill was not disappointed that he was not the primary decision maker in the family. From the time he was married, his wife had assumed the decision-making role, and he was very comfortable with that situation. Having been a nonassertive person, he was comfortable letting his wife bathe and dress him. His level of self-expectation was low, so Bill never expected to resume his previous occupational roles. When he was told what potential he could reach, he stated that he would like to learn how to dress himself with one hand, take a bath independently in the bathtub, and, if at all possible, return to work and drive his car. Bill further stated that before his illness, his leisure activities had been swimming and weight lifting.

Within 12 hours Bill was dressing and bathing himself with minimal assistance. Since the only authority and assertiveness Bill had ever exercised was at work, the occupational therapist suggested that Bill's therapy occur outside the home, on the assumption that he would thereby be more likely to assume an active role in his own treatment as opposed to a passive role in his home.

Because Bill's work required him to walk and to use both hands on a computer terminal, the main obstacle to his returning to work was the left-side paresis. In keeping with the occupational behavior paradigm and the patient's occupational history, weight lifting and swimming were used for the therapeutic process and a private athletic center became the site. Bill assumed responsibility for his progress, and because he was in the company of normal healthy people, his earlier passive resignation to his incapabilities was replaced by confidence that he could return to the mainstream. Bill returned not only to work, but also to enjoying life to its fullest. He was independent in all his occupational roles. Although his wife continued to be the decision-maker at home, he was once again the breadwinner.

CONCLUSION

These two case studies illustrate the application of certain principles of occupational therapy to hospice care. Both patients were encouraged to resume their former roles and lifestyles either by physical adaptation or by devising coping mechanisms to overcome barriers. The entire therapeutic approach was designed around the patient's former patterns of adaptation. Goals and expectations were realistic, and the integrity of both patients was preserved.

Hospice is concerned with the quality of life during the time remaining to the dying patient. Occupational therapy, through its knowledge and understanding of human occupation, can play a significant role in helping the terminally ill patient resume his occupational role and, as such, it has a definite place in facilitating quality of life. Occupational therapy has a unique contribution to make to the terminally ill person because of its focus on the use of time and the significance of time to the person who has little left. The opportunity to use this time creatively and to bring satisfactory closure to the final months, weeks, days of another's life is a contribution of immeasurable importance.

Like any other critically ill or disabled person, the terminally ill patient wants desperately to hope that all is not lost. Referral to a therapist implies that the doctor has hope of improvement, or he would not have sent a therapist. Traditionally, occupational therapists hope to return patients, irrespective of their disability, to full independence or, failing that, hope to provide them with the necessary skills to be as independent and productive as their limitations permit. The occupational therapist, like the physician, and nurse, and social worker working with the terminally ill, must be honest with the patient in regard to the illness and what can be achieved. "In treating the terminally ill cancer patient, an extremely fine line must be drawn between encouraging the patient to try to achieve and become as independent as possible without raising false hopes that cannot be fulfilled by the patient or by the therapist."[3, p. 170] By raising false hopes in order to alleviate the patient's feelings of hopelessness, the ground work will be laid for even greater pain. "You gave me hope and I failed."

People who know they are dying become depressed. They feel they have failed as parent, spouse, or friend, and they feel guilty. These are all painful feelings. Occupational therapy is invaluable in a hospice setting because it focuses the patient's feeling of self-worth on competency to be a productive person. The occupational therapist who re-establishes a sense of worth in the terminally ill cancer patient by maximizing his occupational roles makes a significant contribution to the reduction of the cancer patient's pain.

REFERENCES

1. Tigges K: Looking to the future, Western New York Multiple Sclerosis Annual Conference. Unpublished paper. September 1983.

2. Reilly M: A psychiatric occupational therapy program as a teaching model. *Am J Occup Ther* 1966; XX, 2:61-67.

3. Tigges K: Occupational therapy in hospice. In *Hospice Care: Principles and Practice.* Charles A. Corr, Donna M. Corr, Editors. New York: Springer Publishing Co., 1983.

RELATED READINGS

Tigges K, Holland A: The hospice movement: A time for professional action and commitment, *Brit J Occup* Ther 44: 373-376, 1981.

Tigges K, Sherman L: The treatment of the hospice patient: From occupational history to occupational role. *Am J Occup Ther* 37: 235-238, 1983.

Flanigan K: The art of the possible—occupational therapy in terminal care. *Brit J Occup Ther* 45: 274-276, 1982.

Picard H, Magno J: The role of occupational therapy in hospice care. *Am J Occup Ther* 36: 592-598, 1982.

Twycross R: Principles and practice of pain relief in terminal cancer. In *Hospice Care: Principles and Practice,* Charles A. Corr, Donna M. Corr, Editors. New York: Springer Publishing Co., 1983.

Twycross R: Relief of terminal pain. *Brit Med Journal* 4: 212-214, 1975.

Saunders C: Care of the Dying (series). *Nursing Times* 72; No. 26: 1003-1005; No. 27: 1049-1051; No. 28: 1089-1091; No. 29: 1133-1135; No. 30: 1172-1174; No. 31: 1203-1205; No. 32: 1247-1249, 1976.

Wilkes E, Crowthers A.G.O., and Greaves C.W.K.H.: A different kind of day hospital. *Brit Med Journal* 2: 1053-1056, 1978.

The Schultz Structured Interview for Assessing Upper Extremity Pain

Karen S. Schultz, MS, OTR

ABSTRACT. Trauma and disease processes in the upper extremity frequently cause pain as well as impairment in movement, strength and in function. While perception of pain occurs normally in response to bodily insult, prolonged or severe pain may interfere with attempts to maximize physical function and to return the involved person to optimal occupational role. Whether participating as a member on a medical or vocational rehabilitation team, the occupational therapist must adequately assess the area, nature and behavior of pain prior to providing appropriate intervention and recommendations to other team members. A structured interview to assess pain furnishes the therapist with a format for evaluation that is thorough and methodical. The structure and process of the interview allows the therapist to collect subjective information which can be coupled with objective findings from standard upper extremity evaluation and/or observation of task performance. Data gathered will assist the therapist in discovering the etiology of pain, in evaluating the appropriateness of complaints as they relate to pathology and in making appropriate recommendations about the patient's future work roles.

Pain frequently accompanies injury and chronic disease in the upper extremity. According to Taber's Medical Dictionary,[1] pain is "a sensation in which a person experiences discomfort, distress or suffering due to provocation of sensory nerves." The definition goes on to state that, "In most cases, pain stimuli are harmful to the body and tend to bring about reactions by which the body protects it-

The author received her Master's degree in Occupational Therapy from San Jose State University. She is an Active member of the American Society of Hand Therapists (ASHT) and is a Certified Vocational Evaluator (CVE). In her private practice in Santa Monica, California, she specializes in rehabilitation and evaluation of patients with upper extremity problems.

Acknowledgement to Ronald Melzak for portions of the assessment form.

self.'' Pain is the mechanism by which the body signals that a problem is present, such as inflammation, or that the environment threatens, as when the perception of heat helps the avoidance of serious burn. Thus, the perception of pain is essential for survival.

However, when discomfort remains at extreme levels, it can interfere with the achievement of treatment goals. Attempts to restore optimal movement, balance, endurance and function is impeded. Upper extremity pain may in fact preclude engagement in any productive activity and frequently such a painful individual becomes fixed in a role of "patient."

Whether the occupational therapist participates on the medical team or in vocational rehabilitation efforts, she must have a thorough understanding of the nature of the patient's pain. Such an understanding may be derived from an evaluation focused on upper extremity pain in conjunction with information gleaned from the medical history, from range of motion, strength and sensory evaluations, and from observation of the patient performing various activities. Once the etiology of the pain problem is identified, the therapist can often provide appropriate diagnosis and ameliorate the discomfort. A methodic evaluation may give clues about the appropriateness of the patient's complaints as they relate to his pathology. Finally, an accurate assessment of the behavior of the pain (how and why the pain varies) and of the manner in which pain impacts upon daily function enables the therapist to make recommendations about the patient's future work potential.

During evaluation, the person with upper extremity involvement will often provide the therapist with copious numbers of descriptors of pain and its concomitant effects upon his ability to perform daily tasks. While evaluating and treating patients with hand and upper extremity problems, the author worked as a team member in both the medical and vocational setting. During this time, she recognized a need to better organize data gathered. Subjective information, assembled by a structured interview format, could yield a profile of meaningful data that would supplement objective parts of an evaluation. Frequently an interview alone can paint a picture of the individual comprehensive enough to indicate the nature of a pain problem. At other times, however, objective measures and observations of activity are paired with the interview to support or to refute the subjective information which the patient provides. The synthesis of subjective and objective data often provides a more accurate total picture of function.

DEVELOPMENT OF THE TOOL

Development of the structured interview of upper extremity pain (see Figure 1) began in the Hand Rehabilitation Unit at the University of California at Los Angeles where patients with traumatic injuries and chronic disease received treatment for upper extremity dysfunction. The diagnoses of these patients included replantation, free tissue transfer, tendon repair, transfer and grafting, crush injury, reconstruction of rheumatic disease-related deformities, reflex sympathetic dystrophy, burn and amputation. In addition to standard

PATIENT:
DATE:

schultz upper extremity pain assessment

PAIN TREND

Indicate which word completes the sentences correctly.

	increased	decreased	remained unchanged
Compared to when pain began, it has			
Over the past month, pain has			

Comments:

WHERE IS YOUR PAIN?

On the drawings below, please mark an "X" in the area(s) where you feel pain or abnormal sensation. Next to the "X", write an "S" if the pain is superficial and an "I" if the pain is internal. Write "SI" if the pain is both superficial and internal. Give each area of pain a letter, beginning with "A" then "B" etc.

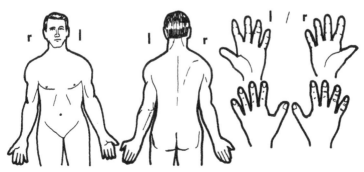

FIGURE 1

evaluations of range of motion, strength and sensation, some way to quantify and categorize subjective complaints was seen as needed in many of the conditions treated. The interview was refined while being used at the Downey Community Hospital Hand Center and Employment Potential Improvement Center as well as in the author's private practice. The populations seen in these settings paralleled those at UCLA. However, also seen were groups of clients who had completed medical management and were participating in physical capacity evaluations and work hardening programs. The content of the interview questions draws from the work of Maitland,[2] Mooney,[3,4] Matheson[5] and Melzack.[6] The evaluations designed by these authors revealed information specific to intensity of pain as well as to the description of the pattern and variance of the pain. However, no evaluation focused on the pain problems specific to upper extremity disorders nor on the impact of pain on a patient's activities of daily living (including self-care, household responsibilities, work and leisure activities) and independence.

PREPARATION FOR THE INTERVIEW

Prior to conducting the pain assessment, the evaluator gathers relevant medical treatment data concerning the evaluee. This material, obtained from medical records and the patient's own reports, includes both the recent and past history. The recent history contains information about diagnosis, nature and date of onset, description of primary dysfunction, the medical management of the dysfunction and the progress from onset until the present. Past history consists of information about any previous traumas or disease processes which may be predisposing factors to the current dysfunction and complaints.

ADMINISTRATION OF THE ASSESSMENT

Prepared with this background information, the therapist evaluates the patient by asking a series of questions following the interview format. The evaluator may read the questions directly from the assessment form or rephrase them. The questions on the assessment have been structured precisely to guide the patient to reveal the types of information desired. It is essential that the evaluator remain in control of the interview; she must make sure the patient provides responses which are directly related to the questions asked and should not accept random or evasive responses. The order of the questions is not crucial, although some sections flow together nicely.

Melzack[6] states that, "Preliminary studies showed that data obtained by allowing a patient to fill out the questionnaire by himself are sometimes unreliable. Patients may fail to read the instructions carefully and miss . . . essential features . . ." To make sure instructions are fully understood by the patient, Melzack advocates that the questions be read aloud to the patient. The evaluator provides clarification of the meaning of a word when the patient does not understand it. The patient selects the answer he deems appropriate. Either the patient or the evaluator may write the answers on the form. Any elaboration provided by the patient is noted in the "comments" section.

THE INTERVIEW FORMAT

The Structured Interview for Assessing Pain in the Upper Extremity, as seen in Figures 1-3, is designed to capture information concerning the area, nature and behaviors of pain in the upper extremity. The components of the assessment are (in this order):

—Pain trend
—Location of pain
—How your pain feels
—Duration of pain
—Intensity of pain
—Pain and time of day
—Pain and sleep
—Causes of increases and decreases in pain
—Activity and pain

Pain Trend

To get an idea of how the pain has changed since onset, the therapist asks if the pain has increased, has decreased or has remained the same. The evaluator then asks about the course of symptoms over the past month prior to evaluation. When either "increased" or

<u>HOW YOUR PAIN FEELS</u>

Please describe as accurately as you can how your pain feels. For each description indicate where on your body that type of pain is felt by using the letters "A", "B" etc. from the drawing on the previous page.

<u>DURATION OF YOUR PAIN</u>

Circle the word which completes the sentence accurately.

My pain is constant
        intermittent
        momentary

Comments:

<u>INTENSITY OF YOUR PAIN</u>

The words and numbers below represent pain of increasing intensity.

ABSENT	MILD	UNCOMFORTABLE	DISTRESSING	SEVERE
1	2	3	4	5

Choose the number of the word which best describes:

___Your pain right now
___Your pain at its least intensity
___Your pain at its maximum intensity
___The worst pain you have ever felt

Comments:

<u>PAIN AND TIME OF DAY</u>

What time of day does your pain begin or increase?

___morning
___afternoon
___evening
___during sleep

Comments:

<u>PAIN AND SLEEP</u>

Please indicate how pain affects your sleep by the checking the accurate word.

	Always	Sometimes	Never
I have difficulty falling asleep			
I need medication to sleep			
I am awakened by pain			
I am able to lie on my painful part			

Average hours of sleep per night:____

Comments:

FIGURE 2

FIGURE 2 cont'd

CAUSES OF INCREASES (+) AND DECREASES (-) IN PAIN LEVEL

Indicate a "+" or a "-" opposite the cause of change in pain level.

Liquor	Vibration	Tension
Medication	Movement*	Loud noises
Heat	Rest	Heavy activity
Cold	Pacing	Light exercise
Damp	Splints/supports	Activity*
Weather change	Proper body mechanics	Position*
Massage	Home modification*	Sleep
Pressure	Workplace modification*	Fatigue
Impact (using hammer)	Task modification*	Use of gloves

*Specify in comments section

Comments:

ACTIVITY AND PAIN

(a)What happens to your pain when you do each of the following tasks?
Please also indicate how long a pain increase lasts if it occurs.
Circle any activity you cannot perform for reasons other than pain.

	No change	Increases			Duration
		a little	moderately	a lot	
1.Use fingers to:					
pick up a coin					
close a safety pin					
use clothing buttons					
2.Use hands to:					
hold eating utensils					
brush teeth					
open jars					
3.Reach to:					
replace a lightbulb					
wash hair					
pick up object off the floor					
4.Push and pull:					
open and close car door					
iron clothes					
vacuum					
mow lawn					
5.Lift:					
trashcan					
groceries					
children					
6.Carry:					
groceries					
suitcase for overnight stay					
purse/briefcase					
7.Twist to:					
wring out a towel					
use a screwdriver					
use a hand can opener					

Comments:

FIGURE 3

FIGURE 3 cont'd

ACTIVITY AND PAIN

(b)Below is a list of activities. Please indicate how pain affects your ability to perform these activities.
You may be able to perform the tasks in the same amnner as you always have.
You may have to slow down and/or change the method of doing the activity.
You may need a break before being able to complete the task.
You may need help from another person or from a piece of equipment or tool.
You may not be able to do it at all.

ACTIVITY	NO CHANGE	SLOW DOWN	CHANGE METHOD	NEED BREAK	NEED HELP	UNABLE
1.Dressing fasteners, shirt, shoes socks, pullover						
2.Food preparation cutting, stirring, opening containers						
3.Self-care bathing, care of teeth of nails and of hair						
4.Home maintenance cleaning, gardening organizing						
5.Communication writing, using phone						
6.Transportation driving, using bus/ subway, riding bike						
7.Hobbies						
8.Sports/recreation						
9.Work job which you had at the time of disability						

Comments:

"decreased" is the response, the therapist should determine if the patient has any ideas about why the status of the pain has changed. For example, the level of the individual's activity may have changed or medication may have been discontinued, thus affecting his pain levels. The information gathered in this section is important for giving the therapist insight into the attitude and outlook of the patient.

Location of Pain

To identify the location(s) of pain, the interviewer asks the patient to indicate where on the extremity pain is felt. To answer, he is asked to mark on the anterior and posterior body diagrams provided on the assessment form. In addition to the body diagrams, large diagrams of both the palmar and dorsal surfaces of the hand are available for marking (see Figure 1). The patient is also asked to indicate whether the pain is experienced deep inside the extremity or superficially.

Specificity in marking is crucial. A person with significant pain complaints should be able to pinpoint the location of discomfort.[7] The absence of such specificity may be one of the first indicators of pain of non-physical etiology. The evaluator should be certain to note vague or inconsistent reports on the site(s) of pain.

Precise identifications of the pain site(s) can give clues to the etiology of the pain. Complaints of discomfort over the digital nerve sites at the distal and of a finger amputation stump may indicate neuroma formation. Reports of radiating pain up the forearm which follow the course of a major nerve may indicate peripheral neuropathy. Complaints of pain which involve the entire upper extremity, the neck, the head, and back may indicate the need for the patient to have a more extensive medical work-up or to undergo a psychological evaluation. Non-physical etiology of pain also becomes a possibility when the patient reports anesthesia in a distribution that does not follow anatomic structures.

Quality of Pain

Melzack and Torgerson[8] studied words used to describe pain experience. They found, "that the word 'pain' refers to an endless variety of qualities that are categorized under a single linguistic label, not to a specific single sensation that varies only in intensity. Each pain has unique qualities. The pain of a toothache is obviously different from that of a pin-prick . . ." These researchers identified three major classes and sixteen subclasses of descriptors. "The classes are: (1) words that describe the *sensory qualities* of the experience in terms of temporal, spatial, pressure, thermal and other properties; (2) words that describe *affective qualities* in terms of tension, fear, and autonomic properties that are part of the pain experience; and (3) *evaluative* words that describe the subjective overall intensity of the total pain experience." (6) Melzack and Torgerson's study also assigned relative intensities to the words in each subclass. Their articles describe the manner in which the choice of words may offer more information to the clinician involved in evaluating and treating patients with pain. It is beyond the scope of this article to elaborate further and the reader is encouraged to review the works of Melzack and Torgerson.

Melzack and Torgerson advocate providing patients with words to describe their pain. They found that the patients were selective and that the word lists saved the patient from having to grope for the words. In the hand clinic, use of the list reduces test administration time.

On the assessment form (see Figure 2), an area is provided for the therapist to write the words which the patient reports as descriptive of his pain. Next to each word the therapist writes the letter from the preceding diagram which corresponds to the area on the patient's body where that type of pain is felt. In this way, the data gained in the previous section on "Location of Pain" combines with data from this section. When the therapist brings together location of pain with quality of pain, she is often better able to identify the cause or nature of pain. A report of "electric pain" in combination with the designation of the site of pain at the site of nerve laceration gives more weight to the impression of neuroma formation as the etiology of pain.

Duration of Pain

The words used in this section are excerpted from Melzack.[6] The data gathered here represents a general idea of the amount of time the patient is involved in the pain experience each day. (See Figure 2)

Intensity of Pain

Using a five point scale and corresponding five word descriptors adapted from Melzack, the evaluator asks the patient to rate his pain at the time of the interview, at its least and at its maximum intensity. He is also asked to rate the worst pain he has ever felt. This data, when combined with that from "Duration of pain" and with observation of the patient yields valuable information. Reports of pain of high intensity and of constant duration may indicate to the evaluator either that the patient is experiencing an extreme amount of discomfort, has the *belief* that he experiences an extreme amount of discomfort, or is attempting to exaggerate the level of discomfort. Often the patient's body language or demeanor will provide clues which help to discriminate which of these three situations pertain. People with extreme pain seldom move quickly nor do they have relaxed posture or animated speech. A patient's demeanor may support or cast doubt upon a high rating of ongoing pain. (see Figure 2)

Pain and Time of Day

To determine what is the pattern of pain over each 24 hour period, the therapist must ask the patient what times during the day pain begins or becomes significant. Those who work with upper extremity patients are accustomed to reports of increased pain in the morning after eight hours of immobilization and in the evening after twelve hours of activity. Complaints of increased perception of pain upon going to bed are the most commonly heard. This is believed to occur primarily because of the lack of competing events and stimuli which would divert the patient's attention from the pain experience during waking hours. Based on the data gathered in this section (especially when it is confirmed by objective observation in a workshop setting), the therapist is better able to make recommendations about work roles to vocational rehabilitation counselors or employers. The therapist can suggest the optimum work shift for an individual or may identify the patient's need for work hardening or reconditioning so he can tolerate longer periods of activity. (see Figure 2)

Pain and Sleep

The therapist asks the patient how pain affects his sleep. If a patient reports that pain is so severe that it interferes with falling asleep or staying asleep, this may indicate a significant pain problem. The evaluator may wish to question further to attempt to determine whether emotional problems or physical problems lie at the root of sleep disturbance. She may find that these two factors combine to interfere with sleep. According to orthopedist F. Thornton,[9] complaints of sharp pain which cause sudden wakening from sleep is consistent with diagnosis of tumor. According to Maitland,[2] the inability to lie on the affected part may indicate a mechanical problem in involved joints. When the patient reports a significant decrease in the number of hours of sleep per night, problems of fatigue and changes in temperament can be anticipated. Observations of low frustration tolerance during any subsequent task performance may be related to interview findings of sleep "deprivation." (see Figure 2)

Causes of Increases and Decreases in Pain Level

The therapist presents the patient with a list of factors which are known to either increase or ameliorate pain. The patient is asked to put a " + " next to the factors which aggravate his pain and a " − " next to those which diminish it. The therapist should validate the information gleaned from this part of the interview during subsequent observation of task performance. Consistency and inconsistency between subjective and objective data should be brought out in the summary of findings of the evaluation.

When the patient reports that he takes medication, the therapist should ask what he takes and how frequently. The occasional use of over-the-counter analgesics has minimal impact on employability and on participation in therapy during the acute stages of injury. The report of consistent reliance on prescription medication for pain control indicates a serious problem.

A patient's 'personal' solutions to pain problems reveal a great deal about the patient, such as his innate common sense and problem solving ability. The information also provides clues to possible task and environmental modifications which may help the individual return more rapidly to productive activity. On occasion a patient will report constant pain of unchanging intensity in preceding sections of the interview and in this section will report that a factor increases or decreases his pain. The therapist should note this conflict in information. She may wish to bring it immediately to the patient's attention or may choose to simply include the finding in the final report. (see Figure 2)

Activity and Pain

This section of the interview consists of two parts, part (a) and part (b). (Figure 3)

Part (a): With the focus on various components of activity, such as reaching and lifting, the therapist asks the patient if and how his pain varies when he attempts various tasks. Sample tasks vary in amount of resistance encountered and/or in the amount of endurance required to perform them. The examples of tasks provided are activities of daily living which generalize well to the work setting.

The patient is also asked to indicate how long a pain increase persists if it occurs. Maitland[2] states, "Irritability is determined by relating the vigor of an activity which causes pain, firstly to the degree of pain which ensues, and then to the length of time taken for this increased pain to subside to its usual level." The patient's description of his degree of irritability should be compared with that seen in observation of performance. If the patient states that very little activity causes considerable pain which takes a long time to subside, the therapist will need to be cautious during the objective work sample and/or physical evaluations that follow the interview. The data from this section aids the therapist to appropriately design and grade the patient's therapy program or the work sample evaluation.

Part (b): While section "a" focuses on how the components of upper extremity function affect the patient's pain level, section "b" focuses on the manner in which pain affects the patient's ability to perform various activities. The interview expands on the classic activities of daily living assessment which includes the categories "independent", "requires assistance" and "unable". Also included are categories which reflect the way a patient might modify a task in order to complete it independently. He might need to slow down, to alter the method of performance or take breaks. The therapist should ask the patient how long his breaks last before he can resume activity and how frequently he must take them.

This data is crucial when the purpose of the evaluation is to assist vocational personnel to return the patient to work. For example, a patient who reports the need for frequent breaks of greater than a minute may have significant difficulty with meeting productivity requirements of a job. On a more positive note, the patient's own task modifications may give the therapist clues about ways to modify work so that the patient may sustain himself in a job for a full work day. The data also reveals areas of difficulty which may require a therapist's intervention to facilitate greater ease of performance or independence in activity.

SUMMARY

The Structured Interview for Assessing Upper Extremity Pain is one component of a complete upper extremity evaluation. Its value lies in its use as a methodical data gathering tool. It organizes information which heretofore has been gathered in a random manner.

The organization makes the information more accessible to the evaluator and therefore facilitates a more comprehensive evaluation. The interview format allows the occupational therapist to be precise and to obtain desired data during the evaluation of highly subjective material.

Inherent in the questions in the Structured Interview is a check and balance system. While each section of the assessment is distinct, some overlap does purposely exist. This allows the therapist to check for consistency in the patient's responses. Both consistency and inconsistency should be noted in the summary of data collected. The author has incorporated copies of the assessment forms in the evaluation report as well as a brief summation of findings in the "Summary and Recommendations" section of the report.

The Structured Interview combines with the expertise of the therapist to generate needed information. Skill is required not only in evaluation and treatment of upper extremity patients but also in administration of the evaluation instrument. As the therapist gains experience in the use of the Structured Interview, the data gathered will become more precise and the ability to summarize from the data will improve.

The sections of the Structured Interview can be combined in various ways. This data synthesis produces an impression of the cause and nature of the patient's pain and of the impact of the pain on the patient's ability to participate in a therapy program or in the work world. With this information, the occupational therapist may support her recommendations for therapeutic intervention or for the type of work appropriate for the patient.

REFERENCES

1. Thomas, CL (editor): *Taber's Cyclopedic Medical Dictionary* (12th edition), Philadelphia: F.A. Davis Co. 1975

2. Maitland, GD: *Peripheral Manipulation* (2nd edition), Boston: Butterworths, 1977

3. Mooney, V, Cairns, D, and Robertson, J: A system for evaluation and treatment of chronic back disability. *West J Med* 124: 370 - 376, 1976

4. Ransford, AO, Cairns, D, Mooney, V: The pain drawing as an aid to the psychologic evaluation of patients with low back pain. *Spine* 1: 127 - 134, 1976

5. Matheson, LN: *Work Capacity Evaluation,* Trabuco Canyon: Rehabilitation Institute of Southern California, 1982

6. Melzack, R: The McGill Pain Questionnaire: Major properties and scoring methods. *Pain* 1: 277 - 299, 1975

7. Lynn, J: personal communication, 1981

8. Melzack, R. and Torgerson, WS: On the language of pain. *Anesthesiology* 34: 50 - 59, 1971

9. Thornton, F: personal communication, 1983

Shoulder Pain in the Patient with Hemiplegia: A Fundamental Concern in Occupational Therapy

Charlotte Gowland, BS, OTR

ABSTRACT. Shoulder pain in the affected upper extremity of patients with hemiplegia is of fundamental concern to occupational therapists who are working for increased independence of patients. The author interviewed several other occupational therapists, reviewed recent literature and completed a survey of charts of 30 patients. The literature and the therapists' responses indicated a higher frequency of pain than the author anticipated. The chart review was completed (1) to determine objectively the frequency of shoulder pain or subluxation in patients with hemiplegia, and (2) to ascertain the use of the upper extremity and the performance of functional activities of those patients who had shoulder pain or subluxation. Although the number in the sample of charts was too small to yield more than an indication of problems, 3 groups patterns emerged based on the differences in functional use of the upper extremity. These 3 patterns of function were compared with findings in the literature. Further study is suggested to assess pain and its responses to occupational therapy, during both the acute and chronic phases of care. The goal of research would be to better predict which patients would develop shoulder pain, thereby helping to prevent long-term complications.

Shoulder pain in the affected arm of patients with hemiplegia is a fundamental concern of occupational therapists who are working for increased independence with patients. Because of finding persistent occurrences of shoulder pain in early stages of recovery of patients with hemiplegia, the author engaged in an informal review of the

Charlotte Gowland is Occupational Therapy Supervisor, Stroke/Neurology, Head Trauma, Orthopedics/Diabetes & Problem Fracture Services at Rancho Los Amigos Hospital, Downey, CA 90242.

why's and how's of this phenomenon as seen in occupational therapy clinics. Accordingly, a simple three-part exploration was conducted, comprised of informal discussions with occupational therapy colleagues, a limited review of literature related to this aspect of hemiplegia rehabilitation, and a sample retrospective review of charts of patients seen by occupational therapists at Rancho Los Amigos Hospital (RLAH) in the past 2 years.

The purpose of this exploration was (1) to determine how common shoulder pain is in this population, (2) to identify the use of the upper extremity in these patients who had shoulder pain or subluxation and (3) to assess their abilities to perform functional activities. In this article pain is used in a broad sense and refers to that which limits motion, decreases use of the UE and interferes with performance of functional activities. This article will identify questions that hopefully will stimulate research on this topic.

OCCUPATIONAL THERAPIST IMPRESSIONS

Based on treatment of patients at RLAH, using early mobility and positioning to prevent shoulder pain, the author's impressions were that shoulder pain in the patient with hemiplegia was seen in only a small percentage of patients. Savinelli[1] supports that thinking when she states that severe shoulder pain is rarely seen if the patient receives early range of motion within the pain-free arc and has proper positioning for reducing subluxation. Other occupational therapists were interviewed to determine their perceptions about shoulder pain in patients with hemiplegia. Their impressions did not support the author's view that shoulder pain was seen in a small number. They felt the frequency was approximately 10% and that the effects of treatment varied. Occupational therapy measures, regardless of type, appeared without specific reason not to influence the pain for some patients. However, the pain in others responded to similar treatment and was resolved within 6 to 8 weeks. The therapists indicated patients with subluxation often did not complain of shoulder pain.

LITERATURE REVIEW

In reviewing pertinent literature, the author found reports of even higher frequencies (12.5-50%) of shoulder pain. Steinbrocker,[2] for example, reports that the shoulder-hand-syndrome (SHS), in which pain in the shoulder is a key symptom, occurs in stroke more frequently than is commonly reported. He states that SHS is often over-looked because the symptoms of the early phases of SHS are re-solved in spontaneous recovery. However, the difficult problems of SHS are recognized over time and often irreversible changes have already occurred. In a study of 139 patients he reports findings to in-dicate that at least 25% of patients were found to be in one of the stages of SHS. Davis[3] reports that the syndrome occurs in 12.5% of patients with hemiplegia whose disabilities were severe enough for an inpatient rehabilitation admission. Finch[4] reports finding SHS in 50% of patients with hemiplegia admitted in a large acute hospital over a four-month period. In identifying symptoms associated with SHS in these patients, she found that 10 of the 20 patients had symp-toms of decreased range of motion, pain, and swelling (SHS stage 1). This limited literature review supports a range of 12.5-50% oc-currence of shoulder pain in patients with hemiplegia. This is a serious complication in this population. Further research is needed to narrow this range.

CHART REVIEW

One continues to ask why the difference in the reported frequen-cies of shoulder pain in patients with hemiplegia. To try to answer the question in another way, shoulder pain of 30 inpatients at RLAH was studied retrospectively. The charts were randomly selected from among those patients treated during the past 2 years. These pa-tients were 18 males and 12 females whose ages ranged from 44 to 77. A larger percentage had right (R) hemiplegia (60%) than had left (L) hemiplegia (33%), and 7% had bilateral involvement. Time between onset and initiation of rehabilitation services was approxi-mately 1 month with the exception of 1 patient studied who was 3 years post cerebral vascular accident when rehabilitation began.

The answers sought in the chart review were: (1) the frequency of shoulder pain or subluxation, and (2) the UE use and performance of functional activities of those who had pain or subluxation. No standardized method was used to measure pain; pain was subjective-ly based on the therapists' observations. The chart review noted pain as documented by the occupational therapists. The intent of the chart review was to determine if there were patterns to the painful shoulder problems for this patient population that might later be studied in depth. Research in this area could benefit clinicians by helping them to predict likely occurrence of pain in future patients.

Such research would thereby also provide information about preventing long-term complications.

Accordingly, the review proceeded as follows with these results. Ten of the thirty patients had shoulder pain or subluxation. The 10 patients who had these problems were reviewed more carefully to identify their UE use and functional abilities. Wilson's[5] categories of UE use described the UE function. Functional abilities encompassed self-care, home, community, and vocational skills. Based on function of the UE three groups emerged. These were (1) a group with *no* UE use (Group A), (2) a group with *minimal* UE use (Group B), and (3) a group with *bilateral* UE use (Group C). (see Figure 1)

GROUP CHARACTERISTICS

Group A consisted of 3 females, 2 with (R) hemiplegia, 1 with (L) hemiplegia, who had no use of the UE. All 3 patients had moderate to severe pain in the shoulder and/or the entire UE. The clinical picture of the UE was of shoulder subluxation, no motion, decreased sensation, increased muscle tone, poor body handling skills, neglect of the involved side, and impaired motor planning. Functional abilities were 'assisted' to 'independent' in feeding, light hygiene, and dressing and 'unable' in the remainder of self-care and home and community skills. Two of the patients had chronic obstructive pulmonary disease and congestive heart failure in addition to their hemiplegia.

Group B consisted of 5 males, 3 with (R) hemiplegia and 2 with (L) hemiplegia who used the involved UE from a 'minimal assist' to a 'minimal active assist'. All had shoulder subluxation but complained of no pain in the shoulder or UE. The clinical picture of the UE was more variable. It ranged from minimal motion with diminished sensation, impaired perception, neglect, and poor body handling skills to motion deviating from pattern, intact sensation, perception, and body handling skills. Functional abilities varied from 'assisted' in self-care to 'totally independent' in all activities of daily living, including being able to work part-time.

Group C consisted of 1 male and 1 female, both with (R) hemiplegia who used the involved UE in bilateral activities. The clinical picture showed 'fair plus' to 'good' strength with some decrease in fine motor skills; sensation was slightly impaired for two-point discrimination, and perceptual skills were intact. Function was 'in-

GROUP	USE	PAIN	CLINICAL PICTURE	FUNCTIONAL ABILITIES
A (3 pts)	No use	Moderate to Severe	Shoulder subluxed Severe involvement in all areas	Assisted to unable in self-care
B (5 pts)	Minimal assist	None	Shoulder subluxed Moderate to minimal involvement	Assisted to independent in ADL
C (2 pts)	Bilateral use	Minimal	Very minimal involvement	Independent in ADL

Groups identified in the review of charts of patients with hemiplegia

Figure 1

dependent' in activities of daily living except activities requiring extremes of shoulder range. One patient had selective use of the involved dominant extremity for fine motor activities upon discharge from the hospital, but 5 months later complained of severe pain in the entire side of his body and edema in the hand. Pain was so severe he had difficulty sleeping at night; he found positioning the UE in a dependent position gave some relief but caused edema. He also had congestive heart failure and had almost stopped using or even moving the UE. The other patient in Group C had minimal to moderate pain in the shoulder that gradually resolved. Functional limitations were primarily related to reaching objects overhead with the involved arm.

DISCUSSION

Although the number of patients in this review is too limited to identify more than obvious pictures of pain and function, the 3 groups did identify some significant trends when attention is focused on use of the UE and the patient's functional abilities. The patterns of each group will be compared with findings in the literature to determine similarities and differences and to identify potentially helpful treatment strategies.

Findings in Group A showed patients with a combination of pain, no use of the UE, severe involvement of the UE and limited functional abilities. These findings matched some of those in Finch's[4] survey of 20 patients in which she attempted to identify factors associated with SHS in patients with hemiplegia. In her study the patients were divided into two groups: (1) those with pain, swelling and decreased range of motion, and (2) those without symptoms. Ten of the twenty had these symptoms. The independent variables of mental status, sensation, speech, range of motion, muscle tone, functional activities, and shoulder subluxation were compared in these 2 groups to determine if there was a pattern of problems. The patterns that emerged were that the group with SHS were more likely to have decreased mental status, diminished sensation, and shoulder subluxation, and require maximal assistance in functional activities as compared to the group without symptoms.

When comparing these findings with Group A of the current chart review, the findings are similar. Finch's findings not only support the trends seen in Group A but help identify significant variables influencing treatment planning and implementation. The implications for treatment are described by Finch. First, Finch states that during the initial stages of recovery, positioning and moving the patient to prevent the development of pain are critical. That includes positioning in both bed and wheelchair, and during transfers. All persons working with such patients need training in handling the patients properly, including paramedics, families, and patients themselves. Patients with decreased mental status need even more special care to assure adequate protection of the involved extremities.

Second, Finch[4] describes early mobility as part of the treatment program. The treatment program at RLAH uses early mobility, including teaching the patient self-range of motion, and involves the whole body using neurodevelopmental principles in therapeutic exercises and activities. Delisa[6] emphasizes this treatment approach by stating that treatment must be aimed at prevention of the adverse effects from immobility in addition to managing the specific deficits caused by the stroke. To achieve limb movement, range of motion must be preserved. Treatment fights against disuse, gravity, muscle imbalance, synergistic patterns and reflexes, all of which contribute to contractures. Delisa further states that this movement is the more important because pain usually accompanies any UE complications.

Patients in Group B of the chart review showed patterns of using the affected extremity as a minimal assist, having no pain, having shoulder subluxation, having minimal to moderate involvement of the UE and being primarily 'assisted' to 'totally independent' in functional ability. This group had a wide range of functional abilities and accompanying UE clinical pictures. The common findings were the use of the affected UE as a minimal assist, no pain, and subluxed shoulders. Finch's[4] study found that shoulder pain and subluxation were combined in the SHS. The author's chart review showed that patients with severe limitations in UE use, pain, and function may have shoulder subluxation; however, patients in Group B did not fit that pattern for subluxation. In other words, shoulder subluxation by itself may not cause pain. This agrees with the input from the occupational therapy colleagues. When looking at treatment for the patient with a subluxed shoulder, both Finch and the RLAH program agree in the use of early mobility, positioning and support. Questions therefore are raised as to why the differences in pain occurred. One additional treatment used at RLAH by physical and occupational therapy to decrease shoulder subluxation is functional electrical stimulation. The effects of this treatment on subluxation are presently being studied.

Patients in Groups B and C gained early as they recovered some use of their affected extremities. Davis speculates that the incidence of SHS may be lower in patients with less severe strokes since they regain movement earlier and thereby gain more functional use of the upper extremities.

Patients in Groups A and C had additional medical problems that could contribute to pain. Steinbrocker[2] indicates pain may be secondary to associated medical conditions such as pulmonary or cardiac diseases. One of the patients in Group C showed dramatic changes in pain 5 months post-rehabilitation and may be suspect of additional medical problems, including another stroke.

UNANSWERED QUESTIONS

Although suggested patterns of problems were identified in this limited review, more questions were raised than answered. Data are desperately needed to enable the clinician to predict which patient will develop shoulder pain and to help him prevent long-term complications. A number of questions emerge for consideration. *First,* what are the elements of shoulder pain? Where is the most frequent focus? When does it occur? Are the same criteria being used by all the authors describing pain? Does pain always fit into one of the categories of SHS? *Second,* what are the long-term effects of shoulder pain? Is it an isolated problem or does it usually occur as part of a complex of problems? *Third,* how does occupational therapy prevent or influence pain? Do early mobility and positioning strategies prevent shoulder pain? What treatment techniques decrease or eliminate shoulder pain once it has occurred? What are the differences in shoulder problems at various time intervals post-stroke? *Fourth,* how do treatment techniques of other professionals interrelate with those used by the occupational therapist? Do any of these treatment techniques prevent shoulder pain if they are initiated immediately post-stroke?

SUMMARY AND CONCLUSIONS

The question of how common shoulder pain is in the population of patients with hemiplegia treated at Rancho Los Amigos Hospital stimulated interviews with fellow therapists, a literature review and a sample chart review. Major differences were found in frequency of pain reported among all three parts of the study.

Literature shows many in rehabilitation are beginning to study the variables that affect the functional abilities of patients with hemiplegia. Some patterns of pain and function are emerging.

Because occupational therapists have a fundamental concern for assisting patients to their highest levels of independence in daily functional activities, only with better understanding of the cause and role of pain in the affected upper extremity can these goals be effectively pursued.

Further investigation is needed if the therapists are to understand whether pain identified during the acute stage of rehabilitation will continue, despite early treatment, into the chronic phase. Also effort must be made to clarify whether or not all pain identified in hemiplegia is part of the shoulder-hand-syndrome.

With answers to questions about pain provided by valid research will come better treatment strategies and increased functional capabilities for patients. Occupational therapists need to be a part of the search for those answers.

REFERENCES

1. Savinelli, R: Therapy evaluation and management of patients with hemiplegia. *Clin Orthop* 131:15-29, 1978
2. Steinbroker, O: The shoulder-hand syndrome: present perspective. *Arch Phys Med Rehabil* 49:388-395, 1968
3. Davis, SW: Shoulder-hand syndrome in a hemiplegic population: a 5-year retrospective study. *Arch Phys Med Rehabil* 58:353-356, 1977
4. Finch, L: Factors associated with shoulder-hand-syndrome in hemiplegia: Clinical survey. *Physiotherapy Canada* 35:3:145-148, 1983
5. Wilson, D: Assessment of the hemiparetic upper extremity: a functional test. *Occ Ther H Care* 1:2, 1984
6. Delisa, JA: Stroke rehabilitation: Part II - Recovery and complications. *Am Fam Physician* 26:6:143-151, 1982

The Role of Occupational Therapy in Back School

Joy White Randolph, MOT, OTR

ABSTRACT. As 'Back Schools' are finding growing acceptance and recognition as a treatment for patients with back pain, occupational therapists are increasingly becoming involved in programming them. Traditionally such schools have been conceived and implemented by physicians and physical therapists. However as the Back School concept is analyzed, need for direct application of the skills and philosophies of the occupational therapy profession is quite evident.

The core of the Back School program emphasizes that patients control back pain ultimately through the appropriate selection of and approach to their daily activities. Traditionally occupational therapists use directed performance in activities of daily living as ways to maximize patients' function. However, before hurling occupational therapists into the Back School setting one must ask "How much understanding of the biomechanics of the spine does the occupational therapist have?" A real 'backbone' understanding is essential in order for one to teach correct posture and body mechanics to persons who need to engage in all sorts of activities of daily living.

An example of the occupational therapist role in two back school formats offered by the North Texas Back Institute is described. Results of follow-up surveys of back school 'graduates' from both programs are briefly reviewed.

Back Schools are a growing entity in the treatment of persons suffering from back pain.[1] Their focus on the idea that a better educated or informed patient is a patient more responsible for his own health finds many supporters. Further, programs help patients to see that passive acceptance of 'magical' pain relieving potions and miraculous curative acts that are found in many places in today's health system are not viable solutions to their problems.

Influencing an individual's health by directing the use of muscles

---

Joy White Randolph is Director of Back School and Occupational Therapy, North Texas Back Institute, 3801 West 15th Street, Suite 100, Plano, TX 75075.

93

and mind together in activities is a basic premise upon which occupational therapy was founded.[2] In back care programs control of
back pain is largely dependent upon the proper selection and the approach one uses, in mind and body, to activities. Consequently, occupational therapists who are specifically trained in understanding
the biomechanics of the spine and have the profession's traditional
'activity' orientation for treatment find themselves at the core for
implementing the Back School concept.

In order to help persons decrease the effects of back pain and the
risks of further injury Back Schools basically strive for 'directed occupation', in both mind and body, of persons suffering from back
pain. Back School students are generally taught how the back normally works, what can go wrong with it in daily function and how to
avoid further injury. Even greater emphasis is placed upon directing
the student's energies toward controlling his back pain.

In today's age of easy access to information through TV, radio
and popular publications, more and more emphasis is being placed
on self-help techniques as answers to improved personal health and
fitness. While no one media source is trying to deceive the public
that the secret to eternal youth has been discovered, at the same time
individuals are learning that much of what influences their health is
in their own hands. Particular emphasis is being placed on various
aspects of aging and how anyone can continue to live a quality lifestyle and still not hasten aging or jeopardize his health.

Health care philosophies as seen in use today by various health
care providers are evolving in much the same way. Those giving
medical services are increasingly speaking of personal responsibility for health maintenance gained through greater understandings of
causes of illness and ways of finding the right care. The Back School
concept evolved when persons applied these same ideas of health
care to the treatment of persons suffering from back pain. The
Swedes and Canadians developed the earliest models followed by
providers in the U.S. who adopted the self-help philosophy in programs in various clinics around the country.[3,4]

The universal theme in Back Schools is to teach the control of
pain.[5] However, the ways in which this is carried out varies considerably from setting to setting.[6] Nonetheless, regardless of differences in approaches final results appear to be quite similar.[7] The
experiences of the Back Schools at the North Texas Back Institute
will be described to demonstrate two approaches to such programming.

INITIAL TREATMENT PLAN

In 1978, the North Texas Back Institute was founded in Plano, Texas by two orthopedic surgeons, Stephen Hochschuler, M.D. and Ralph Rashbaum, M.D. A major service of the Institute from the start was its back school, then called the 'Spinal Care Program'. This was a 12 hour multi-disciplinary program which included both individual evaluation and training of patients and group classes. The disciplines participating, after physician examination and referral to the program, included physical therapy, occupational therapy and clinical psychology. For the program, which extended over a period of several weeks, patients came to the clinic for four visits, each of approximately three hours.

On the first visit, or 'Day One', the patient underwent an individual physical therapy evaluation and was given immediate postural instruction for correct sitting, standing, lying as well as for temporary rest positions. The patient also received an individual occupational therapy evaluation including assessment and recommendations for performance of activities at home, work and play. He also received a body mechanics 'obstacle course' evaluation. During that course which included various activities involving reaching, lifting, pushing and pulling the patient was scored on the percentage of correct body mechanics and postures he used in performing the tasks. Finally, the patient was given an EMG biofeedback screening in which muscle tension of the head, neck, upper body and lower body was charted on a body diagram to produce a profile of resting EMG values as grossly normal or exceeding normal in various severities.

Within a week, on the second visit, or 'Day Two', the patient first attended a 1 1/2 hour class of 5 to 10 patients in which a physical therapist taught them about spinal anatomy, degenerative processes, treatments and procedures commonly prescribed by physicians to minimize back pain. During the second half of the Day Two visit, a clinical psychologist taught the group about the body's psychophysiological responses to pain and stress in the environment.

Within another week the patient returned for 'Day Three' to be in a smaller training class of 3 to 5 patients in which a physical therapist taught about muscles and ligaments generally related to back pain. He further instructed the patients in corrective exercises and gave them general fitness guidelines. During the second half of the visit, an occupational therapist presented material on the damaging effects to the spine of poor posture and body mechanics. She then instructed each group member on proper techniques of posture and body mechanics in common activities. This was done by returning each patient to the obstacle course setting.

The patient finally returned in 2 to 4 weeks for 'Day Four', his last visit. This day included individual physical therapy and occupational therapy re-evaluations and final recommendations for continued exercise and fitness regimes as well as suggestions for selection and modification of home, work and play activities. All patients once more performed on the obstacle course for final testing on their body mechanics and posturing, using a peer group to rate how they did. The clinical psychologist closed the program with a group discussion on basic relaxation techniques and of the choices that individuals each have in trying to control their stress and pain.

In the interim between these four visits patients were instructed to carry out exercises and practice of correct postures in all their daily activities and to note the effects these had on their pain.

RESULTS

How effective was this program? In six month, twelve month and eighteen month follow-up surveys conducted by the author as Program Director, the 'graduates' were polled by mail and phone for their subjective assessments of the results and value of the program. Patients were asked specifically for their retrospective assessments of their status 'before' and 'after' the program. A total of 465 surveys were mailed and 38% responded either by written or phone replies. Demographics of respondents indicate they were 45% male, 55% female. Their ages were from 25 to 65 with an average age of 41 years.

Respondents classified the duration and severity of their pain in various ways, including the following: 37% said their back pain lasted for less than six months prior to attending the program; 21% reported having pain for from six months to one year; 13% reported one to three years of pain prior to attending the program; and 29% reported having pain for longer than three years. Fifty-seven percent of those responding had never been hospitalized for their back pain before attending the program.

Responses on post-course condition indicated decreased frequencies and intensities of pain after the program and significant changes in attitudes and understandings about their own needs. Probably these two factors lead to the patients' responses of having improved confidence about approaching activities and a sense of improved control over their pain. As a final result, 93% of those who responded to the survey indicated they would recommend the program to others. (See Table 1)

In addition to these mailed surveys, 189 patients were asked to evaluate the program as they concluded the four visits. This group was about half and half, male and female with an average age of thirty-eight years. Two questions that were asked yielded significant and helpful information regarding improvements in patients' conditions and about which program content was most helpful. (See Figures 1 and 2)

Even with such positive results, many insurance carriers still did not accept the program as necessary or valid as treatment for back conditions. Consequently they refused to pay for the service. Accordingly the North Texas Back Institute changed its back school and general services formats in an attempt to still provide the services but in a way that would reduce costs to patients.

CURRENT BACK SCHOOL PLAN

In August, 1982, the twelve hour Spinal Care Program was condensed to a four hour group educational program called the 'Back School'. Optional outpatient occupational therapy, physical therapy

TABLE 1

SPINAL CARE PROGRAM SURVEY RESULTS

ITEM	BEFORE PROGRAM	AFTER PROGRAM
Pain frequency and intensity	47% constant pain 51% frequent or occasional pain	84% nonexistent or less frequent pain 78% less intense pain
Attitude towards dealing with back pain	66% with postive attitude	97% with positive attitude
Activity approach	39% approached activities with confidence	77% approached activities with confidence
Understanding of their back problem	33% understood their back problem	95% understood their back problem
Ability to control pain	2% felt in control of their back pain	52% felt in control of their back pain

SPINAL CARE PROGRAM

DAY FOUR PATIENT RESPONSES

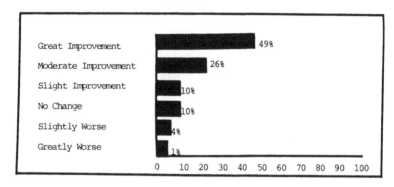

FIGURE 1

Patient Assessment of Their Condition

SPINAL CARE PROGRAM

DAY FOUR PATIENT REPONSES

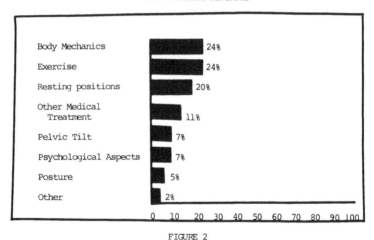

FIGURE 2

Patient Assessment of What Helped Their Condition

and clinical psychology individual services were expanded. At that time, the Institute also moved to a larger, better equipped facility with significantly increased personnel. Many programming changes ensued but for the purposes of this discussion only the changes in the Back School program will be described.

The Back School became one four-hour visit to the clinic, or two two-hour visits, for group education, discussion and participation in various exercises and activity routines. Groups in the School vary from 8 to 15 patients.

The first hour taught by a physical therapist or occupational therapist covers the anatomy of the spine, degenerative processes, first aid and other discussion of modalities, techniques and treatment procedures common for relieving back pain. A plastic model of the spinal column as well as charts, diagrams and illustrations are used as visual aids to supplement teaching. Discussion by patients of their experiences with various modalities and treatments is encouraged.

The second hour of the program is taught by a physical therapist and covers the roles of muscles and ligaments that affect the lower back. All patients are encouraged to participate in performing simple maintenance exercises for the back. General fitness and recreation guidelines are also discussed.

The third hour of the Back School program taught by an occupational therapist covers proper posture and body mechanics in ordinary daily activities. Disc pressure changes with body position and spinal structural stress with poor body positioning are highlighted. Patients perform various activities of daily living to illustrate proper positioning techniques. Mirrored walls, reactions from other patients and of the instructor give the performer feedback on his ways of using his body.

The last hour of the program is lead by a clinical psychologist to begin a discussion of the nature of stress and its causes and to identify methods for stress regulation. Emphasis is placed on the power of each individual's thoughts, attitudes and choices in controlling the risks of back pain.

RESULTS

A six month follow-up, conducted by the author with Jeannette Obal, OTS yielded positive results similar to those from the Spinal Care Program. Fifty-nine or 29.5% of the surveys mailed were returned with written responses. Again respondents were almost evenly divided male and female with an average age of 41 years. Since the North Texas Back Institute is located in a suburb north of Dallas it is not surprising that the respondents from this upper-middle class area showed an average length of formal education of 14.4 years; 39.7% classified their work as sedentary. (See Tables 2 and 3)

Respondents classified the duration and severity of their pain in various ways including the following: 75% denied having had back surgery; 20% claimed to have had one surgical episode; 5% claimed two or more surgeries. Seventeen percent said their back pain had lasted more than one year; 19% reported one to two years of pain; 13% reported two to three years of pain and 26% reported more than 10 years of pain. (See Table 4)

TABLE 2

HIGHEST EDUCATIONAL LEVEL COMPLETED

Grade	N	%
9	3	5.4
10	0	---
11	1	1.8
12	11	19.6
13	5	8.9
14	8	14.3
15	3	5.4
16	15	26.8
17	4	7.1
18	6	10.7
No grade reported	3	---

SOURCE: J. Obal. "A Descriptive Study of the Back School Program at the North Texas Back Institute". M.O.T. Professional Project, Texas Woman's University, 1983. Table 2.

TABLE 3

DESCRIPTION OF WORK CLASSIFICATION

Work Classification	N	%
Sedentary	23	39.7
Light	13	22.4
Medium	17	29.3
Heavy	3	5.2
Very Heavy	2	3.4
No class reported	1	---

SOURCE: J. Obal. "A Descriptive Study of the Back School Program at the North Texas Back Institute". M.O.T. Professional Project, Texas Woman's University, 1983. Table 3.

TABLE 4

BACK SCHOOL SURVEY RESULTS

ITEM	BEFORE PROGRAM	AFTER PROGRAM
Pain frequency	57% constant 21% frequent 21% occasional 0% no pain	16% constant 25% frequent 48% occasional 11% no pain
Pain Intensity	60% severe 34% moderate 6% slightly aggravating 0% no pain	9% severe 45% moderate 31% slightly aggravating 15% no pain

Understanding of their
   back problem
	43% understood their
	   back problem
		97% understood
		   their back
		   problem

It should be noted however that many of the Back School patients, including these respondents, also had received one or more of the individual outpatient services of physical therapy, occupational therapy or clinical psychology. Further studies therefore appear necessary to identify the effectiveness of the Back School program as separate from the possible carry-over effects from other treatment. Most patients, however, have agreed that the Back School as a service is worth its low cost of $85.00 even though some insurance companies still ignore this educational program as a viable form of treatment.

CONCLUSION

Statistics show that "low back pain is the most common cause of Workmen's Compensation payments in the United States and the most common cause of low productivity due to inability to work."[8] As the medical community strives to deal more efficiently and effectively with this large patient population the occupational therapist cannot overlook her vital role in the treatment of patients with back pain. One major role has been described in Back School programming in which occupational therapists give training in the correct performance of activities of daily living to patients seeking to control their back pain. Occupational therapists who are adequately trained in the biomechanics of the spine can appropriately direct and implement activity-focused Back School programs. The time is now.

REFERENCES

1. Attix E A, Tate M A: Low Back School: A Conservative Method for the Treatment of Low Back Pain. *J Miss State Med Assoc* 20: 4-9, 1979.

2. Hopkins H L: An Historical Perspective on Occupational Therapy. In *Willard and Spackman's Occupational Therapy*, Sixth Edition, Hopkins and Smith, Editors. Philadelphia: J B Lippincott Company, 1983, pp 3-20.

3. Anderson G: "LBP - Swedish and U.S. Experience". Paper presented at the *Industrial Low Back Pain* conference, Jeffersonville, Vermont 7 October 1983.

4. Hall H: *The Back Doctor,* New York: McGraw-Hill Book Co., 1980.

5. Attix E A Nichols J: Establishing a Low Back School. *South Med J* 74: 327-331.

6. Kennedy B, Forssell M A, Hall H, Mattmiller A W: International Approaches to Education in Back Care. *Physiotherapy* 66: 108-122.

7. Hochschuler S: "Back School: Analysis of a 4 Hour Program as Compared to a 12 Hour Program". Paper presented at the *International Society for the Study of the Lumbar Spine,* Cambridge, England 8 April 1983.

8. Nordby E J: Epidemiology and Diagnosis in Low Back Injury. *Occup Health Saf* 50: 38-42.

The Use of Biofeedback Techniques in Occupational Therapy for Persons with Chronic Pain

Shelley R. Rogers, OTR
Julie Shuer, MA, OTR
Susan Herzig, MA, OTR

ABSTRACT. The use of biofeedback in occupational therapy to aid the person with chronic pain in the resumption of his daily functional activities is discussed. The chronic pain syndrome and how it disrupts performance of activities is examined, as well as occupational therapy strategies for assessment and treatment using biofeedback, and indications for evaluating treatment outcomes. The authors assume readers have basic familiarity with biofeedback theory, equipment and its operation.

The person experiencing chronic pain who is referred to occupational therapy typically associates activity with his pain and therefore has experienced major lifestyle changes. For this individual the anticipation of pain during and after activity causes anxiety and this disrupts his functional abilities. Such a patient may have to discontinue working, may become dependent on family members for the performance of activities of daily living, or may become socially isolated, all of which events are devastating to role performance.

The goal of occupational therapy using biofeedback for the patient with chronic pain is to enable him to perform functional daily activities without anxiety and without the anticipation of activity-

Shelley R. Rogers is a partner with Julie Shuer in the Los Angeles based private practice known as Occupational Therapy Services. Susan Herzig is in private practice in occupational therapy in San Francisco, California.

induced pain. Occupational therapy in this mode focuses on altering pain behaviors rather than on reducing the pain itself.

THE CHRONIC PAIN PROBLEM

The chronic pain syndrome lasting six months or longer involves not only the primary pain problem, but also the patient's perception of the pain, his respondent pain behaviors and postures, and autonomic nervous system habituation. An individual's perception or anticipation of pain elicits pain behaviors and defensive bracing postures. Pain behaviors include: (1) rapid shallow breathing. (2) sudden withdrawal from sensory stimuli that are perceived as threatening or noxious (touch, noise, temperature changes) and (3) anxiety. Bracing postures include: (1) co-contraction of proximal muscles, (2) decreased spinal and trunk mobility, (3) increased cervical kyphosis, and (4) increased lumbar lordosis. The maintenance of these behaviors and defensive bracing postures causes autonomic nervous system habituation. As a result the patient tends to perceive *all* activity as pain producing and consequently avoids any activity.

Occupational therapy using biofeedback along with other more traditional treatment methods intervenes in the patient's pain cycle by normalizing autonomic nervous system habituation during the performance of activities. The sympathetic and parasympathetic branches of the autonomic nervous system usually function in equilibrium in order to maintain the body's homeostasis. Autonomic nervous system habituation is the disruption of this equilibrium. One of the many physiological changes that takes place when parasympathetic functions predominate is the shift in one's respiration to slow, deep diaphragmatic breathing. This occurs normally during relaxation. Conversely, predominance of sympathetic functions results in shallow, rapid, suppressed respiration. For the normal person this happens during any anxiety-provoking situation.

Most patients with chronic pain demonstrate sympathetic habituation with rapid, shallow respiration, sudden withdrawal from touch, cold hands and feet, constant perspiration and agitation. With parasympathetic habituation, which occurs less frequently with pain, the chronic pain patient experiences inactivity, depression and decreased affect and interest. Patients of either group are candidates for occupational therapy using biofeedback training because their responses to activity in either case are of sympathetic overarousal.

INTERVENTION

The objective of occupational therapy using biofeedback then is to teach the patient with chronic pain to mobilize his suppressed para-sympathetic function during activities. This enables him to use normal breathing responses in activities that affect him along a continuum from arousal to relaxation. Teaching the patient alternative breathing patterns provides him a means of self-regulation, both in stressful situations and during his regular activities.

Assessment

Occupational therapy intervention with the chronic pain patient begins with assessment of functional abilities related to work, rest and leisure, as well as in performance of self-care and of social role responsibilities before and since the onset of pain. Second, trunk and upper extremity strength, range of motion and functional mobility are evaluated. Third, information about the origins of the pain, the patterns of pain and current methods of pain control are obtained by the therapist through interview with the patient. Major questions include:

1. What is the cause and location of the original pain and how was it treated?
2. What was the progression of the pain in terms of time and location?
3. When does the pain occur?
4. Which activities aggravate the pain?
5. Does the intensity of the pain change when the patient feels anxious, upset, agitated or relaxed?
6. Where is the specific location of the pain at this time?
7. Does the patient use drugs, home remedies such as heat, massage, jacuzzi or whirlpool baths; professional services such as relaxation therapy, traction, Transcutaneous Nerve Stimulation, or psychiatric intervention?

Fourth, bracing postures are noted as described above. The patient may demonstrate these habitual postures in numerous positions and activities, e.g., standing, sitting and during locomotion. Finally, baseline electromyometric readings of the scaleni, upper trapezius and diaphragmatic musculature are made with biofeedback monitors.

Treatment

In order to enable the patient to perform daily activities without anxiety and without the anticipation of activity-induced pain, the occupational therapist using biofeedback strategies teaches the patient a five-step sequence designed to elicit and maintain relaxation and deep breathing.

To begin biofeedback training two electromyometers are placed, one on top of the other, and positioned at the patient's eye level. The top machine monitors diaphragmatic musculature which is to be facilitated, while the bottom machine monitors the neck accessory muscles (scaleni) which are to be inhibited. The instrument that monitors diaphragmatic activity will also monitor cardiac electrical impulses (artifact) which will appear as rhythmic fluctuations on the monitor needle.

The objective of the first phase of biofeedback training is to help the patient increase deep breathing by providing auditory feedback from the monitor to reinforce his diaphragmatic function. The patient lies supine with the upper torso elevated to 45°. Upon sufficient diaphragmatic inhalation the monitor shows an increase in the level of baseline fluctuation of 1 to 2.5 microvolts (mv). Additional deep pressure feedback may be provided with a three pound sandbag placed over the patient's abdomen. As the patient increases diaphragmatic breathing the therapist should reinforce the 'feelings' by asking the patient to identify cues of relaxation such as feelings of warmth, heaviness or dizziness. Neck accessory muscles are not monitored at this time.

During the second phase of training the patient sits upright with the back and upper extremities supported, and through trial and error, while deep breathing, attempts to inhibit neck accessory muscle activity below 5 mv. Reinforcement is provided by a decrease in auditory and visual feedback from the monitor. Diaphragmatic activity is not monitored at this time.

In the third phase of training the patient, still deep breathing and sitting upright with the back supported and the upper extremities unsupported, attempts to balance neck accessory muscle and diaphragmatic activity within appropriate ranges on the monitors. Auditory feedback is provided to the less easily regulated muscles, usually the scaleni. The transition to functional activities begins as the patient attempts to balance tension in neck accessory muscles and diaphragmatic breathing during speech. Speaking exercises progress from counting out loud to repeating the names of significant others and finally to conversation. The exercises can be graded from a whisper to normal voice volume.

The fourth phase of training involves the performance of functional activities with biofeedback. Sitting in a chair without back support, the patient performs activities such as typing, simulated driving or a craft, such as macramé. This type of functional upper extremity activity normally increases neck accessory muscle tension. Successful inhibition of neck accessory muscles occurs when the patient is able to return the monitor to a baseline of 5 mv within 5 seconds after cessation of activity.

The fifth step of training is initiated with the patient maintaining monitored equilibrium between neck accessory muscle and diaphragmatic functions. The electrodes are then disconnected and the patient performs modified sensory motor activities without feedback. Sensory motor activities such as doing active range of motion movement and trunk rotation, moving in and out of two and four point kneeling positions, rocking, rolling and crawling are used because they provide stimulation which may arouse the patient's anxiety. These activities are continued until the patient begins to show signs of sympathetic arousal, i.e., shallow breathing, perspiration or flushing. Electrodes are then reattached. The time necessary for the patient to resume appropriate breathing patterns indicates the degree of successful carryover.

OUTCOMES

Progress and final outcomes depend of course on the severity of the patient's problem. Persons who have a relatively short history of pain demonstrate immediate success with altering their breathing patterns during activity. Those who have had a longer pain history may require numerous sessions before they can change breathing patterns and perform activities without arousing anxiety.

Treatment outcomes can be measured by the patient's increasing awareness of his pain behaviors and the consequent reduction of these behaviors when he mobilizes parasympathetic responses. Initially, the patient may report that he felt more relaxed and pain free after treatment but later in the day experienced increased pain. This occurs because following the initial reduction in pain the return perception of pain is greater. Improvement from this status occurs when the patient reports that pain is either less frequent or of less intensity after treatment. The next indication of progress is that the patient is able to anticipate the onset of pain by his awareness of increasing pain behaviors.

Finally in anticipation of pain, the patient is able to elicit at will the breathing patterns that correlate with relaxation. At this point the patient should be capable of maintaining appropriate breathing patterns while performing all activities of daily living. Upon discharge the patient will be able to manage his pain problem while maintaining optimal levels of activity.

SUMMARY

Occupational therapists concerned with helping patients to improve performance of activities of daily living have a real role with persons whose functional abilities are impaired or lost due to chronic pain.

Along with traditional techniques involving the use of activities employed with such patients, biofeedback can be a valuable tool to assist patients in achieving pain-free functional behaviors. These are achieved through monitored learning of relaxed postures and deep breathing patterns that both reduce pain and remove the anxieties associated with activity.

Once patients have learned these responses they can indeed carry them over at will into the performance of all daily activities essentially free of pain.

RELATED READINGS

Abildness AH: *Biofeedback Strategies,* Rockville, MD: American Occupational Therapy Association, 1982.

Barber J, Adrian C *Psychological Approaches to the Management of Pain,* New York: Brunner/Mazel, 1982.

Taylor LP, *Electromyometric Feedback Therapy,* Los Angeles: Biofeedback and Advanced Therapy Institute, 1981.

Thomas CL, *Taber's Encyclopedic Medical Dictionary.* Philadelphia: FA Davis Co, 1973.

The Use of Assertiveness Training with Chronic Pain Patients

Linda Lloyd Zelik, OTR

ABSTRACT. This paper describes one way that occupational therapy participates in a multidisciplinary program for chronic pain management. Assertiveness training as a means of acquiring improved communication skills is presented as one of the techniques used in reducing the emotional stress associated with pain. In addition, some of the other problems associated with the chronic pain syndrome are discussed along with occupational therapy's role in teaching assertiveness. Both the content of the assertion course and teaching examples are presented along with examples from patient participation. Although the assertiveness training has resulted in positive feedback and acceptance from patients, further study is needed to validate the results.

Chronic pain is a complex problem which often affects persons both physically and emotionally. Many find it results in a tremendous upheaval in their lives including disruption of life roles, strained relationships with family and friends, isolation and often times decreased self-concept and self-esteem. These problems are compounded when there is the all too frequent addiction to pain medication.[1-3]

In the multidisciplinary chronic pain management program at Daniel Freeman Marina Hospital, the teaching of life skill tech-

Linda Lloyd Zelik is staff therapist, Daniel Freeman Marina Hospital Pain Management Program, Marina del Rey, California. Previously she worked as a COTA in acute physical disabilities' treatment programs.

The author gratefully acknowledges Becky Thatcher Bell, OTR for her work in originating the assertiveness portion of the chronic pain program, and Jeanette Workman, OTR, Director Occupational Therapy at Daniel Freeman Memorial Hospital for her support and assistance in this work. Special thanks go to my husband, Joseph Zelik, Ph.D., and to Kathy Tracy, RPT for their support and editorial assistance with this article. Also, the author thanks Irene Vega for her typing assistance.

109

niques is utilized in order to increase the patient's awareness and control over his life and his pain. A crucial component of this approach is stress management.[4] Occupational therapy offers assertiveness training as one important technique for decreasing stress through acquiring effective communication techniques.[5,6]

The objective of this article is to describe the rationale for teaching assertive communication to patients with chronic pain or disease and to show why occupational therapy is an appropriate discipline to teach assertiveness. The body of the paper consists of a discussion of assertiveness and its benefits, as well as how the concepts and skills are presented to the patients within this program. The author hopes thereby to stimulate interest in further study and research on this topic so that its use can be validated scientifically. Another desired result is to generate interest among occupational therapists in the use of assertiveness training within other settings such as with psychiatric patients, chronic disease patients, and in preventive health programs.

Before beginning the discussion it is important to provide a basic definition of assertiveness as used in this program. *Assertiveness* is effective communication, that is, being able to listen and to express oneself in an open, honest and direct way. It involves speaking up for one's rights and needs without infringing on the rights of others. Being assertive encourages one to take charge of his own life in order to set and achieve life goals.[6,7]

PROBLEMS ASSOCIATED WITH THE CHRONIC PAIN SYNDROME

Chronic pain can lead to total disruption of a person's lifestyle. Very often one with chronic pain feels like a victim, not only of the pain but of the medical profession as well. He may feel helpless and hopeless, and such feelings tend to decrease self-confidence and self-esteem. Frequently his communication and the focus on his life centers around the pain.[2] It is not uncommon to see a patient use his pain through such pain behaviors as limping or complaining in order to avoid honest communication. Interpersonal relationships with family or friends are often strained because a person with chronic pain frequently is irritable and possesses limited coping skills.[1,3] Life goals may be put aside or forgotten because one no longer feels in control of his life.[2]

RATIONALE FOR USING ASSERTIVENESS TRAINING

Much research has been done in recent years linking stress and disease. Emotional stress has been found to increase the intensity of pain, to help maintain the chronic pain cycle, and in some cases to actually cause pain or disease.[4,8,9] Long term illness tends to foster effects such as isolation, negative self-concept, depression, and anxiety.[2] It is understandable that in such circumstances communication skills might be diminished and, in some cases, such loss might have been a predisposing factor in the chronic pain or illness.[4] Assertiveness training is seen as a way to help patients break the stress/pain cycle by decreasing their emotional stress and lack of control in their environments caused by ineffectual communication.[10] Assertive behavior may also result in long term stress reduction because, when used, it encourages others to respond to the person with increased respect and fairness.[11]

OCCUPATIONAL THERAPY'S ROLE

The philosophy that directs occupational therapy practice mandates that the therapist take into account the biological, psychological and social aspects of human development as they affect daily function. The therapist is concerned with promoting independence and competence within life roles, assisting persons to gain mastery over their environment.[12] Effective communication is one very important skill in the development of competence and mastery over environment.[13] In 1979 the American Occupational Therapy Association published the Uniform Terminology System for Reporting Occupational Therapy Services.[14] In the section related to psychological/emotional living skills treatment it discusses "situational coping". This is described as ". . . skill and performance in handling stress and dealing with problems and changes in a manner which is functional for self and others." Some of the components included are: interactions with others, both dyadic and group; directing and redirecting energy in order to overcome problems; and assuming responsibility for self and consequences of actions. These are all behaviors which can be enhanced by the understanding and practical application of assertive communication. Based on this concern for successful coping in life roles, occupational therapy thus may be considered an appropriate discipline to teach assertiveness, particularly in long term rehabilitation or psychiatric settings.

BACKGROUND

The overall goals of the pain management at Daniel Freeman Marina Hospital are to teach patients how to cope more effectively despite some degree of ongoing pain and to return to a more normal and meaningful lifestyle without the need for pain medication. The multidisciplinary team conducting the program includes a neurologist, a psychologist, an occupational therapist, a social worker and psychiatric nurses. The overall treatment approach is operant conditioning with a strong emphasis on teaching self-help methods for achieving a healthy and balanced lifestyle. In addition to the assertion training, various other stress reducing techniques are utilized which include relaxation, bio-feedback and pacing. This is all incorporated into a five week intensive inpatient program which is structured and primarily uses the 'group approach'. The patient population consists of adults who come to the program with a wide variety of diagnoses. These include spinal and low back injuries, migraine headaches, post herpetic neuralgia and pain that is secondary to other diseases such as arthritis or diabetes. Patients are admitted in groups of three or four; there are two in-patient groups and one out-patient group which run simultaneously.

Occupational therapy sessions comprise a large portion of the patient's program. These sessions include:

1. Daily work tolerance groups using craft activities primarily for increasing standing and/or sitting endurance while improving work skills.
2. Three to four education classes per week covering topics such as body mechanics, energy conservation, assertion, pacing, scheduling, balance of work, rest and play, development of leisure activities and goal setting.
3. Weekly outings and leisure skill groups for reorienting patients to the community and for increasing their "fun levels".[2]
4. Individual sessions with the patients to address special needs, such as work role counseling.

ADVANTAGES OF ASSERTIVENESS

Some of the advantages of being assertive, particularly for persons with chronic pain, are that such behavior:

1. Allows expression of emotions and needs rather than internalizing them, which can cause stress.
2. Encourages honest and direct communication in lieu of maladaptive coping behaviors. For instance, patients may use pain or illness to avoid difficult or unpleasant dealings with family, friends and co-workers.[1]
3. Allows the use of verbal problem solving to reduce or eliminate certain unsuccessful situations.[11,15]
4. Provides an option not to be manipulated by circumstances or other people.[10]
5. Tends to foster increased self-confidence and self-esteem.[15]
6. Tends to facilitate the transformation of decisions and plans into actions since assertive behavior is goal directed.[17]

DESCRIPTION OF ASSERTIVENESS CLASSES

The patients receive six hours of classroom instruction in assertiveness which includes theory, discussion and practice through role playing. Assertiveness training is introduced in the second week of the five week program and continues for approximately two weeks. The patients are expected to participate through class discussions, role playing and homework assignments. Each patient is also given handouts which include a class outline, practice worksheets, and a bibliography of suggested additional reading.

The overall goal of the assertiveness training is for each patient to be able to express/assert himself when he wants to, rather than reverting to previous ineffective coping behaviors.[17]

The course objectives for patients are:

1. To help patients understand how stress in their lives can adversely affect their pain status and how assertive behavior can decrease this stress.
2. To teach the concepts of assertive communication and to enable each patient to describe and demonstrate through role-

playing practice specific techniques he can use in various life situations.
3. To assist each patient to recognize and identify his own assertive and non-assertive behaviors and to transfer the assertive techniques learned to his actual life situations.

The initial class is an introduction to assertiveness in which definitions as well as course objectives are presented. The class discussion includes reasons for and benefits of teaching assertiveness to persons with chronic pain.

To compliment the definition of assertiveness mentioned earlier in this paper, two additional definitions are needed for clarification. Being *passive* is not communicating honestly or openly, thereby allowing one's own rights, needs or desires to be violated.[7] Being *aggressive,* on the other hand, is not considering the needs or feelings of others while trying to fulfill one's desires or goals.[18]

It is stressed to the patients that all persons, at times, can be either passive, assertive, or aggressive, depending on the circumstances. The training in assertiveness is presented as a means to increase options for more effective communication, particularly in stressful situations.

The second hour of instruction deals with the relationship of stress to pain. The physiological effects of emotionally stressful situations are identified and explained. Assertive communication is referred to as a coping mechanism. It is explained that although there is no way to eliminate stress in our society today, verbal problem solving can be utilized in many instances to decrease or eliminate stress.

Non-verbal communication (body language) techniques are explored in the third class. The meaning of words can be changed dramatically depending on such things as tone of voice, eye contact, hand gestures and facial expression.[15] As an example, the simple command, "Close the door", is stated to the patients in three different ways, assertively, passively, and aggressively. The patients practice role playing these techniques with an enjoyable game called "Assert Now".[19] Utilizing this non-threatening format helps patients become more comfortable with role playing. The game involves rolling a die to determine if the message on a role card is to be acted out passively, assertively, or aggressively. The therapist plays along with the group of 3 or 4 patients. Initially, the cards are comical and help put the players at ease. For example, "After 43

years together you still can't pronounce my name right, it's Pat!''.
Later, more realistic situations are used like, "The bank has no
record of a night deposit you made, and your checks are bouncing
all over town. What do you say?'' The patients are given a homework assignment of observing someone's body language and describing it in the next class.

The fourth class consists of exploring ways to improve communication skills, both of listening and speaking. The importance of good
listening skills is emphasized and practiced. One technique used is to
have each patient briefly describe an incident from his life to another
patient. The other patient then re-tells the incident to test the accura-
cy of his listening. Specific techniques for improved speaking skills
are also covered.[5, 11, 15] The objective is to keep communication lines
open in difficult or stressful situations and to defuse potential destructive conflicts.[16] Examples are presented and role-play practice
follows. Patients are asked to practice the listening exercise with
someone as 'homework'.

Frequently chronic pain patients have difficulty with anger, and
particularly in giving themselves 'permission' to be angry. The fifth
class session deals with teaching patients to look at anger as a
natural, normal, and healthy emotion. Specific techniques are given
to enable them to practice expression of this feeling. These include
saying words that express anger, such as: "I'm ____ (mad, angry,
frustrated, etc.).'' They are given formulas with examples to help
express their anger in a constructive way. For instance, "I feel
(feeling word) when you *(clear, direct statement of problem)*. In the
future I would like *(desired change).* '' Patients are asked to take
problem situations in their own lives and to verbally role-play them
in class using this and other formulas which are presented. One patient who had some communication problems in her marriage completed the formula in class with, "I feel frustrated and foolish when
you don't listen to me. In the future I would like you to give me
some kind of feedback to let me know you are listening.'' When the
patient presented this statement to her husband, they were able to
discuss and resolve a problem.

Discussion of conflict resolution is also included in this hour. The
patients are taught some basic techniques for turning a potentially
destructive 'fight' into one where both parties can win, at least to
some degree. A few of the basic principles discussed are: (1) having
a clear understanding of the problem and mutual goals, (2) avoiding
accusatory "you" statements, such as "You always . . .'', and (3)

attacking the problem, not the person.[17] Video-tape examples of such situations are presented, and patients practice role-playing of anticipated situations from their own lives.

The last session of the six hour course presents specific techniques for dealing with a variety of stressful situations one may encounter. These include handling criticism, dealing with aggressive sales people, and knowing when and how to suggest compromise solutions.[6,11] Further role playing practice is done using these and other stressful situations that patients expect to encounter after discharge. Patients are asked to give feedback on each other's performances during these role-playing practices. Video recording is used to illustrate additional examples of assertive techniques as well as to enable the patients to observe themselves in these role-playing situations. Patients are encouraged to continued developing their assertive skills after discharge from the program through additional reading and by participating in assertion courses offered in the community.

The program content presented here is only a synopsis and is not intended to provide enough information to teach assertiveness. If one wishes to develop such a course, additional reading from the reference list is necessary, and further study through participation in seminars or classes is recommended.

PROGRAM RESULTS AND CASE EXAMPLES

To date no formal study has been done to measure the degree to which patients become more assertive after completing the program. Almost all of the patients, however, have given positive feedback regarding the assertiveness program. Also, patients frequently have reported back to the staff about specific incidents that they handled better because of applying assertion techniques. An example of this is a man who had suffered from migraine headaches most of his life. Six months after graduating from the program he stated: ''I never used to say anything when my kids would upset me or make me angry. I used to hold everything inside, but now I get things off my chest . . . and I feel much better for it, too!''

Many chronic pain patients tend to behave more toward the passive end of the passive-aggressive continuum, particularly at the beginning of the program. One example of this is a woman who resented having to get up early every day to fix breakfast for her husband. Although this activity increased her back pain, she felt obligated to do it. As one of her class homework assignments she stated these feelings to her husband and was delighted to see how receptive he was to her needs and how willing he was to prepare his own breakfast. This paved the way for better communication in general and less tension between them.

Less frequently chronic pain patients display aggressive behaviors. The disadvantages of being aggressive tend to center around the guilt and/or strained relationships that result. An example of aggressive behavior was a man with a teenage son who reported tensions between them. When the boy did not do as he was ordered, the father would explode with an angry outburst. After the assertiveness class he reported taking a different tack. When his son did not perform an agreed upon yard chore, he stated calmly, "I'm disappointed because you had promised to do it." The son responded with an apology and proceeded to do an excellent job of the chore. Not only was this patient surprised at how much more effective the assertive approach had been, but also noted a significant decrease in tension at home and a corresponding decrease in his pain.

CONCLUSIONS

Assertiveness training appears to be one effective technique for helping chronic pain patients gain control over their pain. Upon completing the Daniel Freeman Marina program, the patients usually report a significant decrease in their pain levels and increased abilities in handling emotionally stressful situations. By this time staff also have observed patients to be generally more effective in communicating their needs and feelings. The patients' overall feedback about the assertiveness training has been very favorable. It should be noted that in a multidisciplinary and comprehensive program such as this one, no one modality or teaching strategy can be singled out as being directly responsible for enabling a patient to gain control over his pain. The success of this program has been achieved by the combination of inputs from an entire team who work together for the best interest of each patient.

It is the desire of the author to stimulate increased interest in assertiveness training so that it will be used more extensively as an occupational therapy modality and so that studies will be initiated to confirm its effectiveness.

REFERENCES

1. Shanfield S B, Killingsworth R N: The psychiatric aspects of pain. *Psychiatric Annals* 7:1, 11-19, 1977

2. Bresler D E: *Free Yourself From Pain.* New York: Wallaby Books, 1979

3. Flower A, et al: An occupational therapy program for chronic back pain. *Am J Occup Ther* 35: 243-248, 1981

4. Pelletier K R: *Mind as Healer Mind as Slayer.* New York: Dell Publishing Co., 1977

5. Alberti R E, Emmons M L: *Your Perfect Right: A Guide to Assertive Behavior.* San Luis Obispo, Calif: Impact, 1970

6. Fensterheim H, Baer, J: *Don't Say Yes When You Want to Say No.* New York: Dell Publishing Co., 1975

7. Jakubowski-Spector P: Facilitating the growth of women through assertive training. *The Counseling Psychologist* 4:1, 75-86, 1973

8. McQuade W, Aikman A: *Stress.* New York: E.P. Dutton & Co., Inc., 1974

9. Benson H: *The Mind/Body Effect.* New York: Berkley Publishing Corporation, 1979

10. Dyer W: *Pulling Your Own Strings.* New York: Hearst Corp., 1978

11. Smith M J: *When I Say No, I Feel Guilty.* New York: The Dial Press, 1975

12. Hopkins H L, Smith H D: *Willard and Spackman's Occupational Therapy,* 5th Edition. Philadelphia: J.B. Lippincott Company 1978, p. 27-28

13. Lazarus A: *Multimodal Behavior Therapy.* New York: Springer Publishing Co., 1976

14. AOTA Commission on Practice: *Uniform Terminology System for Reporting Occupational Therapy Services.* Rockville, Md: AOTA, Inc., 1979

15. Alberti R E, Emmons M L: *Stand Up, Speak Out, Talk Back!* San Luis Obispo, Calif.: Impact Publishers, Inc., 1970

16. Back G R, Wyden P: *The Intimate Enemy.* New York: William Morrow & Co., 1968

17. The Professional Staff Association: *Occupational Therapy in the Care of Spinal Pain Patients Rancho Los Amigos Hospital.* Downey, Calif: The Professional Staff Association of the Rancho Los Amigos Hospital, Inc., 1980, p. 4.29-4.42

18. Baer J: *How to be an Assertive (not aggressive) Woman.* New York: The New American Library, Inc., 1976

19. Greenly L: *Assert Now* (game). P.O. Box 922, Ukiah, Calif. 95487

RELATED READINGS

Dyer W: *The Sky's the Limit.* New York: Simon & Schuster (Pocket Books), 1980.

Phelps S, Austin M: *The Assertive Woman,* San Luis Obispo, CA: Impact Press, 1975.

Seabury D: *The Art of Selfishness.* New York: Julian Messner, Inc., 1937.

Sternback R A: *How Can I Learn To Live With Pain When It Hurts So Much?* Second Edition. La Jolla, Calif: Scripps Clinic and Research Foundation, 1983.

The Growth of the Hospice Movement:
A Role for Occupational Therapy

Pamela Brown, COTA, MA

ABSTRACT. This paper traces the history of the hospice movement, its present status and its projection for growth. It looks at hospices in the United States and in Great Britain, particularly examining the kinds of pain associated with terminal illness, and the alleviation thereof. It compares the philosophy of hospice with the philosophy of occupational therapy and concludes with hope for the future of occupational therapy as an integral part of this humane program which provides palliative and supportive care for terminally ill patients and their families.

Given the similarity between the philosophy of hospice and that of occupational therapy, it is the author's intent to review the history of the hospice movement using limited examples of past and present hospice models, to examine the several concerns of patients who are cared for in such systems, particularly to look at pain, its kinds, its effects and its management. With that overview, the present and potential roles for occupational therapy personnel in hospice can be better understood and appreciated.

Hospice philosophy, though variously defined, focuses, as does the philosophy of occupational therapy, on the quality of life. "To enable the patient to live life as fully as possible with as many options as possible."[1] "By skilled and experienced awareness of a patient's symptoms and feelings, to help that patient to live to the limit of his or her potential in physical strength, in mental and emotional capacity and in social relationships."[2]

The common thread in hospice and occupational therapy is quali-

Pamela Brown was educated in England and in the United States. She is presently consultant to nursing homes in Southern California, and Substitute Instructor in the Occupational Therapy Department, Los Angeles City College, Los Angeles, CA.

ty of life. Each uses a wholistic approach and each fosters self ac-
tualisation.

A DEFINITION

The Latin word "hospes" means host (receiver of guests.) From
this root word comes hospice, defined as a shelter or lodging for
travelers, children or the destitute.[3] In the United States it has been
defined as the relatively new interdisciplinary health care service for
the terminally ill.[4] There are at present some 1200 hospice programs
in the United States.[4] They are of various kinds.

Residential hospice provides inpatient acute care. Home hospice,
sometimes called hospice in the home, or, in Britain, domiciliary
care, provides routine home care or continuous home care (intensive nursing) in the patient's home. Respite care is temporary inpatient care for varying periods of time for the stabilisation of drugs
and/or to allow the primary care givers a rest from the immediate
responsibility and thereby enable them to resume the ongoing care
of a terminally ill person.

The difference between hospice and a hospital is significant. The
hospital treats a patient with the goal of eventual cure. A patient is
admitted into the hospice program with the understanding that death
is imminent. Hospice programs are designed to prepare the patient
and his family for this death, recognizing the role of the family as
caregivers and recognizing also their need to be involved in care
planning and to receive counseling and other services.

A LOOK AT THE BEGINNINGS—BRITAIN

The medieval hospice was a way station which sheltered and fed
pilgrims and travelers until they were ready to continue their
journey, and cared for the sick and wounded. A Catholic order, the
Irish Sisters of Charity opened Our Lady's Hospice in Dublin, Ire-
land, in 1846, and St. Joseph's Hospice (which is still treating the
terminally ill) in London, England, in 1902. These two hospices
cared for many long term patients but made those who were 'going
on the journey from life to death' their special concern.

In 1967 St. Christopher's, a residential hospice, opened in Sydenham, England. It has 62 beds. St. Christopher's was the first re-

search and teaching hospice and epitomizes "an alternative program that brings maximum comfort and dignity to those who are terminally ill."[5]

St. Christopher's was purpose built. That is, it was designed and built to be a hospice. A five storied building with many windows it stands in a garden in a London suburb. The windows are important, not only as proven antidotes for depression, but because a terminal cancer patient left the founder, Dr. Cicely Saunders, a thousand dollars "for a window in your home." It was the first bequest.

A visit to St. Christopher's is not easily forgotten. The atmosphere itself is welcoming. No sterile ambiance, no gleaming machines, no bells or buzzers are perceived. In the garden are flowers, trees, a fountain, visitors, patients—and children. In the building are vibrant and colorful paintings. Each bed has a colorful afghan or quilt and several pillows. Each bed has curtains that can be drawn around it. Personal possessions abound. One wing of the building is a residence for elderly (well) persons, and also on the grounds is a nursery for children of staff members.

Founded by a Trust and operated by the National Health Service the J. Arthur Rank House in Cambridge, England opened its doors in 1981. This residential hospice of 25 beds is situated on the garden grounds of a 45 bed long term care hospital for the elderly. The hospice and hospital share occupational therapy services. Here respite care is featured in various patterns, some patients going home each weekend, some admitted for several days at regular intervals, and some becoming in-patients for a period of several weeks. Because home hospice care is so demanding of the care givers this respite care service is especially valuable. In the Rank House newsletter of July, 1983, the Medical Director says "Every day a call comes from a general practitioner or hospital doctor asking for help with a family which has come to the end of its resources. It is very encouraging to see how skilled nursing care and the calm atmosphere of the hospice relieve the tensions in both the patient and their relatives. Once their symptoms are relieved many return home, and the family manages once again, supported by the knowledge that the hospice is there if it is needed."[6]

This hospice offers many normal living amenities to patients and their families. The visitors' kitchen is kept well equipped and stocked by volunteers and both patients and families are encouraged to indulge in a snack or to cook a special or favorite meal. There is a small beauty shop with a visiting beautician, and a bedroom where a family member may stay overnight. A strong volunteer group raises $400 to $740 a month which can be spent at the discretion of the hospice team.

An example of home hospice in Britain is Hospicare in Exeter, England. Housed in the National Health Service building, it has been in operation for less than two years. With a staff of five plus community support of advisors and volunteers this hospice serves twenty five to thirty families at a time and offers follow up services as well as bereavement care and counseling. Hospicare prefers to increase their home care capacity as they expand rather than starting in-patient services. Hospicare is one of the approximately fifty five home hospice programs in Britain.[7]

IN THE UNITED STATES

Perhaps the best known adaptation of the British residential hospice in the United States is the 44 bed Connecticut Hospice Inc. Incorporated in November of 1971 it was the first hospice in this country other than the religious institutions dedicated to the care of the incurably ill. This hospice, as St. Christopher's in England, was purpose built and the buildings personify and augment the hospice philosophy.

A home care hospice that has received media attention is the Hospice of Marin in San Rafael, California which is licensed as a home health care agency by the State of California. It was founded in November 1975 and operates from an office suite. Hospice of Marin gets considerable community support, has its own thrift shop to augment funds and plans soon to open a residence of eight to ten beds for respite care. Marin is fortunate to get 19% of its funding from the San Francisco Foundation. As a licensed home health care agency it has also, since October 1980, received reimbursement from Medicare for eligible patients.

The home hospice of the Verdugo Hills Visiting Nurse Association in Glendale, California is typical of home hospices. It has been in existence four years and is part of a home health care agency. Its services are provided by a small professional staff, an extended team of para-professionals and over a hundred volunteers, each of whom is interviewed prior to being accepted for training and assignment. Personal interviews and special training of volunteers is standard procedure in hospice programs both in Britain and the United

States, as is the 24 hour "hot line" which is an integral part of home hospice programs. This is a vital service and is rarely abused. As proof of growing community support Verdugo Hills has recently been approached by a local business wishing to sponsor a hospice benefit.

COMPARISON

These various programs, in Great Britain and in the United States, share a common approach as well as the philosophy of hospice. The caretakers are included as part of the unit of care; psychosocial and spiritual needs are addressed as well as the physical; bereavement counseling is given; there is strong volunteer participation; there is consistent exchange of information within the care team; there is community support and there is mutual and professional support of care team members on a regular schedule and most important, the patient's needs are central to all care.

While occupational therapy is not yet found in all hospices in either country there is growing evidence that it is being seen increasingly as a vital discipline for this kind of care.

KINDS OF PAIN IN TERMINAL ILLNESS

When a patient first comes under hospice care he often has feelings of being abandoned and isolated. Friends, even family, not knowing how to relate or what to say, sometimes withdraw, sometimes falsely reassure. A final rejection felt by some cancer patients is the still sometimes held belief that the illness could be infectious so demonstrations of love and affection are withheld. A terminally ill patient has had to abandon his occupational roles, be they as spouse, parent, worker, retiree. Medical personnel, faced with inevitable death seem to lose interest.

Leo Tolstoy, speaking for the character Ivan Ilych who is dying of cancer says; "At certain moments after prolonged suffering he wished most of all . . . for someone to pity him as a sick child is pitied . . . (he) wanted to weep, wanted to be petted and cried over . . . This falsity around him and within him did more than anything else to poison his last days."[8] Emotional pain is as overwhelming to suffer, and therefore as important to treat as is physical pain. Like Ivan Ilych many patients may be unable to express this pain and it may present itself as withdrawal, anger, depression or physical pain. While it often cannot be eliminated it must be acknowledged.[9] Sometimes, since emotional pain and physical pain are so interwoven comforting care techniques used in hospice care—strategically placed pillows, massage, application of heat or ice can bring surcease. Sometimes the work of the caregivers is "to absorb some of the rage."[10]

Since 1965 the hospice movement has given much attention to the nature of terminal pain, the better understanding of pain in general, and on more effective treatment techniques. Alongside this has come a revival of the old concept of 'a good death.'[11] "The chronic pain of terminal disease," says Dr. T. S. West of St. Christopher's Hospice, "without meaning or purpose, and getting worse rather than better is a very different thing from the acute pains of normal life . . ."[10] For cancer patients any new or additional physical pain carries with it the ominous threat of physical deterioration.

In hospice care drugs are administered to block the useless chronic pain of terminal disease. Drugs are given, not as needed (PRN) but before the pain breaks through. When medication is taken regularly around the clock the cycle of pain, anxiety, pain, depression, pain does not get started, and the patient escapes the feeling of being dependent on the drug and on the person who administers it.[12] The analgesic now most commonly used both in Britain and in the United States is a morphine, compazine and cherry syrup combination known as Hospice Mix.

None of the hospices studied by this author reported problems with narcotic dependence though some patients have reported that, prior to hospice care, they had known doctors to express this concern. The consensus of patients and care takers was that psychological dependence was more likely to occur when drugs were given PRN, and the literature bears this out. Physical addiction was not seen by these terminal patients as a relevant problem.

Concurrent with traditional medical care hospice teams address themselves to the lessening of pain wholistically. Provision of a pleasant environment with familiar possessions, the presence of caring people offering quality time, the gift of touch, the provision of favorite records or tapes, books or television programs, assistance with attaining a degree of independence, granting choices will decrease feelings of isolation and help to minimize pain. Hospice philosophy has accepted that we live our lives on three levels. To treat the physical, mental or spiritual as separate one from the other is contrary to hospice belief system. It is equally contrary to the philosophy of occupational therapy.

EFFECTS ON CAREGIVERS

Because of the obvious emotional strain of caring for those who are terminally ill hospices make provision for the care of health team members. At the heart of the hospice program there must be a strengthening of these care givers so that they are able to go on caring. The outside world sometimes lacks understanding of and appreciation for those who care but cannot cure. A hospice volunteer when interviewed said: "It is a privilege to go to the brink with another human being, but I have to have surcease. I need the support meetings." Both residential and home care programs regularly hold staff support meetings. Sometimes these are aided by an outside facilitator or by a staff psychiatrist or psychotherapist consultant. Because of the potentials for stress staff and volunteers are screened very carefully before they are asked to give service. Support meetings are usually obligatory. Dr. Cicely Saunders says: "Hospice work is very taxing . . . We in this work are always somehow missing an outer layer of skin and we must take care to renew ourselves."[13]

Hospice team members may experience feelings of isolation from friends and family because of their intense involvement with patients who are dying. One British team worker said: "A friend of mine was admitted here, and though my family tried to be supportive only my co-workers really understood what I was going through." Working in a hospice program is a growth experience and growth brings pain. A Glendale volunteer said: "I have learned so much about myself. I am a controlling person. I wanted people to die a good death by my standards and I have learned that my way is not the only way, the right way." As in occupational therapy, in hospice patients must set their own goals.

ROLE OF OCCUPATIONAL THERAPY IN HOSPICE

The end of a life is as significant as the beginning or the middle and goal setting is equally important. Assisting patients regain some autonomy and to take responsibility for their own lives is perhaps even more significant when there is little time left. Occupational therapists have worked with hospice patients who had become dependent on the care giver for feeding, bathing and dressing and enabled them to achieve a degree of independence in every area. Tigges and Sherman cite a case study of a cancer patient who made significant gains in self care and resumption of work role in the last few months of his life.[14]

Arts and crafts activities can reassure a patient of his ability to function on some level, and hand made gifts enable a role reversal wherein the patient becomes the giver. Journal keeping, writing of family history, autobiography and reminiscing are more than diversional activities. (One terminally ill patient of the author's acquaintance kept a "Nothing Book" in which she recorded an event or thought each day. It became a treasured legacy.)

Poetry has a surprising power to heal. It is interesting to note that Asclepius, the god of healing, was the son of Apollo, god of poetry. Kenneth Koch's book on teaching poetry writing in a nursing home explores this modality.[15]

CONCLUSION

The more a person can do for himself and the more interests he has up until the very last moment of his life the better the quality of that life—and death.

With this emphasis on the quality of life, the dignity and comfort of the individual, and his need for making choices the hospice model presents an ideal setting for the skills of occupational therapy.

REFERENCES

1. Hospice of Marin, San Rafael, California, and Hospice of Verdugo Hills Visiting Nurse Association, Glendale, California.

2. Saunders, Cicely, "Hospice Care," Reprint. *Am J Med,* November 1978.

3. Morris, William, editor. *"The American Heritage Dictionary of the English Language".* New York: American Heritage, 1970.

4. Halamandaris, Val J, Editor. "Proposed Hospice Regulations Previewed". *Caring.* June 1983, Vol. 2, No. 6. Washington D.C.: National Association for Home Care.

5. Conversation with Paul Hultquist, Executive Director, Hospice Organisation of Southern California, October 1983.

6. *Friends of Arthur Rank House and Brookfields Hospital Newsletter,* Cambridge, July 1983.

7. *Directory of Hospices,* St. Christopher's Hospice, London, England. July/August 1983.

8. Tolstoy, Leo. *The Death of Ivan Ilych & Other Stories.* New York: New American Library, 1960.

9. Earnshaw-Smith, Elisabeth. "Emotional Pain in Dying Patients & their Families." Reprint. *Nursing Times* November 3, 1982. Basingstoke, England: Macmillan, 1982.

10. West, T.S. "Hospice Care for a Dying Patient and his Family." Reprint. Text of a paper given at the *First International Conference on Patient Counseling,* Amsterdam, the Netherlands. April 1976.

11. Saunders, Cicely. "Care of the Dying." Reprint. *World Health,* magazine of the World Health Organisation, 1976.

12. Lack, Sylvia. *A Hospice Handbook.* Hamilton, M. & Reid, G. editors. Michigan: Eerdmans, 1980.

13. Saunders, Cicely. *Interview filmed by the British Broadcasting Corporation.* Screened at St. Christopher's Hospice Sydenham, England, June 1983.

14. Tigges, Kent Nelson & Sherman, Lawrence Mark. "The Treatment of the Hospice Patient: From Occupational History to Occupational Role." *Am J Occ Ther* 37:235-238, 1983.

15. Koch, Kenneth. I Never Told Anybody. *"Teaching Poetry Writing in a Nursing Home."* New York: Vintage Books, Random House, 1978.

What Every Therapist Should Know: Hazards in the Clinic

Michele Watkins, OTR
Lawanna Drake, OTR
Suzanne May, OTR

Many occupational therapists work daily in clinics where potentially hazardous materials are used. Therapists are also exposed to particular stress factors which often cause health problems. This essay examines chemical hazards and stress and how these may affect the therapist. Its ideas stem from a study conducted by the authors. (See Note)

When one uses a product daily without apparent consequences, it is often easy to forget the potential hazards that product could cause. The therapist may be unaware of the side effects of the chemicals in products or fail to realize how chemicals enter the body.

CHEMICALS

Chemicals may enter the body in several ways. They may be absorbed through the skin by air spaces in the hair follicles to the sebaceous glands and gland cells. They may also enter the body in the

Michele Watkins is employed as occupational therapist by the St. Tammany Parish School System in Louisiana. Lawanna Drake is a staff occupational therapist at Lakeshore Rehabilitation Hospital, Birmingham, AL. Suzanne May is both in private practice and employed by PRNS Home Health Care in Maryville, TN.

form of gases, vapors, or mists which tend to pass through the lungs and into the bloodstream to be distributed throughout the body.[1] Dust and fumes also enter the body through inhalation as in the case of fiber dusts. There are several things to keep in mind when examining health hazards that could be caused by chemicals: the concentration of the chemical, how frequently it is used, and the ventilation in the area of use. Also observe carefully any precautions listed on labels or in instructional materials.

An important issue to address in considering chemicals as health hazards is the effects of lead on the human body, in particular on the reproductive system. Often found in occupational therapy clinics are some materials containing lead such as slip, certain types of ceramic glazes and pyrometric cones, some silkscreen inks, and particular brands of enamel paints. In addition to causing anemia, lead directly crosses the placenta of pregnant women and may cause mutations in the fetus. It can also cause menstrual disorders, loss of sex drive, atrophy of testes and possible sperm alteration. Formal studies for the passage of lead through the placenta were begun in the 1930's on rats. Researchers found an increase in kidney weight and liver size, a decrease in femur weight, cleft palate, and hydronephrosis in the babies of female rats exposed to lead. The second generation had a 50 percent increase in mortality rate, stunted growth and sterility.[2] The information is worthwhile to note since the majority of occupational therapists are females who may often work during pregnancy.

Art Supplies

Due to limited space in this presentation only the more commonly used materials will be discussed. Art supplies such as oil paints and turpentine contain chemicals that often cause irritated mucous membranes, headaches, inability to concentrate, gastrointestinal disturbances or skin irritation. In a survey done by the authors, glue was the most commonly used supply with 56 percent of the occupational therapy clinics using it 'frequently'. Acrylic glues contain methylmethoacrylate which irritates the skin. Its vapors may cause nausea, loss of appetite, headaches or decreased blood pressure.

Spray fixatives are detrimental to one's health not only because of the chemicals present in them, but also because their fine mists travel long distances before settling; therefore, they can penetrate deeper into the lungs. The spray may also contain a large quantity of solvent. Some fixatives contain acrylic resin, aromatic hydrocarbons, aliphatic hydrocarbons or toluse. These chemicals may cause dizziness, nausea, incoordination, loss of appetite, anemia, skin irritation or edema.

Some grout sealers contain petroleum distillates, types of solvents that may cause drowsiness, dizziness or skin irritation. If ingested, this chemical could cause pulmonary edema. Chronic inhalation of large amounts may cause peripheral neuritis. It is also a fire hazard when exposed to heat and should be stored in a well-ventilated, cool, dark place. Grout and tile cleaners contain phosphoric acid which is a chronic local irritant.

Leather Supplies

Certain brands of leather dyes and dye solvents contain denatured ethyl alcohol which may irritate the eyes and mucous membranes. Exposure to high concentrations for periods longer than one hour may cause stupor and drowsiness. Exposure to high concentrations may also cause headaches, loss of appetite or an inability to concentrate. Neat Lac Finisher contains toluol which may cause drowsiness or skin irritation. Exposure to moderate concentrations may cause headaches, nausea, loss of appetite or incoordination. Neat Lac Thinner contains petroleum distillates and methanol. Methanol is a type of alcohol solvent that may cause dizziness, intoxication, blurred vision and possible liver and kidney damage if one is exposed to high concentrations. If swallowed, methanol could cause blindness and even death. It is recommended that products containing methanol be used only in well ventilated areas.

Woodworking Supplies

Certain wood stains contain mineral spirits which may cause conjunctivitis, nose and throat irritation, skin irritation, headaches, dizziness, drowsiness, mental confusion, cough, dyspnea, bronchitis, nausea, vomiting, nervousness, blurred vision, ataxia or even convulsions. In this survey, wood stains were the most frequently used substances in the woodworking category. Oil stains such as Phelan's Penetrating Oil Stain contain resins, dye, benzol and naptha. Poisoning by benzol most commonly occurs through the inhalation of its vapors.[3] Benzol may cause drowsiness, dizziness or skin irritation. Chronic poisoning from the cumulative effects of exposure to small amounts can destroy bone marrow and lead to the loss of red and white blood cells and sometimes leukemia. The ingestion of naptha causes a burning sensation, vomiting, diarrhea and drowsiness.

Lacquer and paint thinners were another popular supply used by facilities surveyed. Some thinners contain petroleum distillates and aromatic hydrocarbons while others contain methanol. Health problems related to the use of these chemicals include: severe coughing, irritated mucous membranes, eye irritation, blurred vision, eyes sensitive to light and edema.

Splinting Materials

Most of the facilities surveyed stocked some types of splinting materials. Orthotic cements may contain various chemicals. Kay Splint Cement contains methyl chloride whereas BeOK Orthotic Cement contains toluol, acetone and hexane. Hexane is a type of petroleum distillate that may produce narcosis and skin and lung irritation when one is exposed to large amounts. If ingested, it could cause pulmonary edema and possibly death. Hexane may also cause peripheral neuritis and possible paralysis from chronic inhalation of large amounts. Velcro adhesive contains acetone and methy-ethyl-ketone. Methyl-ethyl-ketone is a solvent that can produce narcosis, eye and mucous membrane irritation and defatting of the skin. This chemical is considered more toxic than acetone and is very flammable.

CERAMIC SUPPLIES

If the occupational therapy clinic has a kiln, good ventilation is vitally important. Not only do some ceramic supplies contain lead, but ceramic clays contain silica which if inhaled or ingested may cause shortness of breath, decreased chest expansion, and an increased susceptibility to infections. When fired, ceramic clays emit 70 pounds particulate/ton of input during the drying process.[3] The most hazardous operations occur when mixing clay dust and when breaking up dry grog.

Some non-firing glazes contain toluene which may cause narcosis or skin irritation. Exposure to large concentrations may produce headaches, nausea, loss of appetite or impairment of coordination. Glazes containing lead are usually clearly marked on the labels.

Both Duncan and Amaco produce some glazes that contain fritted lead compounds or silicious materials.

FIBERS

Fifty percent of the facilities surveyed used yarns 'frequently' in the treatment setting. Fiber dusts from jute cord, cotton, wool or synthetic yarns may cause respiratory irritation and sometimes cause allergies to fiber dusts.

STRESS

Ten stress factors for occupational therapists were identified in responses from 104 occupational therapy clinics across the United States. The work-related stressors receiving the highest attention were continuing education, pressure to improve patient treatment, disappointment in lack of patient progress and concern over legal responsibilities. These can all be speculatively linked to fear of failing professionally. Fear of failing, according to Schmidt, is the source most commonly linked to stress.[4]

The second most common source of stress cited in Schmidt's study was the emotional and physical toll that long hours and professional demands made upon the human body. Therapists working eight hours a day under a heavy patient load who spend more than five hours on their feet fit this category. Selye[5] confirms this point by stating that bodily demands and homeostasis act as stressors.

Stress may increase for the therapist who also is providing treatment on her own time after work hours. According to a study by Cooper and Marshall[6] this practice hinders the individual's ability to adapt to job stress, as it limits free time and can physically overtax the body. According to Tanner[7] a good private life is essential in balancing the stress of work.

The feeling of adequacy is important emotionally for reaching high levels of productivity. Feeling adequate comes largely from how others perceive us to be. If a superior, peer or patient has a personality conflict with a therapist it may cause feelings of inadequacy. These same feelings can also be linked to lack of progress in one's patients. Stress occurs when one's own and others' perceptions of what one ought to be do not match who one really is.[8]

Reactions to Stress

Bodily reactions to stress can vary greatly in their intensity and seriousness. These reactions are due partially to one's predisposition or conditioning to different stressors and to the inability to adapt properly.

The three most common reactions to stress found among those in occupational therapy clinics were fatigue, headaches and muscular aches. These aches and fatigue are partially due to long periods of muscle contractions triggered by stress. If stress continues, the coping with stressful stimuli can lower resistance to disease.[9] Depression is also a stress-linked symptom which is common in over-achieving individuals. Occupational therapists are placed in this category as they tend to 'try to do it all'.

SUMMARY

Because the subject of safety in the occupational therapy clinic is such a broad topic, all hazards, such as equipment safety, infection and structural conditions, could not be addressed in this essay. The intent however is to increase the therapist's awareness of potential health hazards in the clinical setting, thus helping her to create a more pleasant, safe environment for herself and fellow therapists as well as for patients.

NOTE

This essay was developed from a study conducted by the authors as undergraduates at the University of Alabama in Birmingham in which they attempted to identify the chemical and stressful hazards encountered in occupational therapy clinics and how the health of occupational therapists is affected by them.

A questionnaire developed for the study was sent to 300 Occupational Therapy Departments in the United States. One-hundred and four working occupational therapists responded.

Although the results of the research failed to reveal actual evidence linking the ill health of clinicians to chemicals in their work settings, the implications for safe use of materials are noteworthy. The stress section of the questionnaire revealed 10 areas of stress encountered by therapists which can lead to various bodily reactions. Further information on the study and questionnaire can be obtained from the authors.

REFERENCES

1. Patty FA: *Industrial hygiene and toxicology* (2nd rev. ed., Vol 1), New York, 1958.
2. Infante PF, Wagoner JK: *Effects of lead on reproduction. Proceedings Conference on Women and the Workplace,* Washington, D.C., 1976.
3. Sax NI: *Dangerous properties of industrial materials* (4th ed.), New York: Van Nostrand Reinhold Company, 1975.
4. Schmidt WH: Basic concepts of organizational stress causes problems (Papers presented at conference of UCLA Institute of Industrial Relations and the National Institute for Occupational Safety and Health, Los Angeles, November, 1977) *American statistical index,* 1979, Microfiche No. 4248-78.
5. Selye H: *The stress of life* (Rev. ed.) New York: McGraw Hill, 1975.
6. Cooper CL, Marshall J: Occupational sources of stress: a review of the literature relating to coronary heart disease and mental ill health (Paper presented at the conference of UCLA Institute of Industrial Relations and the National Institute for Occupational Safety and Health, Los Angeles, November, 1977) *American statistical index,* 1979, Microfiche No. 4248-78.
7. Tanner O: *Stress* (Rev. ed.) Alexandria: Time Life Books, 1979.
8. Coleman JC: *Abnormal psychology and modern life* (Rev. ed.), Glenview: Scott Foresman and Co., 1976.
9. Holmes TH, Masuda M: Psychosomatic syndrome. *Psychology Today,* April 1972, pp. 71-72; 106.